Inspiring Motivation in Children and Youth

Inspiring Motivation in Children and Youth: How to Nurture Environments for Learning explores motivation and its crucial role in promoting well-being in the classroom and life beyond school. It will help all those who work with children and youth to understand and improve their motivation, and to create nurturing environments for younger people.

David Bergin provides a highly accessible exploration of key research, examining the ways children's goals, self-efficacy, self-determination, and feelings of being cared for affect their motivation as well as their desire to learn more about themselves and the world. This essential guide also addresses influences of competition, diversity, prejudice, and discrimination on motivation. The book provides a comprehensive look at the importance of instilling motivation at this critical age, highlighting the benefits through real-life examples and anecdotes. Illustrated with stories from diverse contexts, the author provides practical advice on how to use goals effectively, help children feel competent, autonomous, and like they belong.

Inspiring Motivation in Children and Youth is for any student looking to excel in a psychological, educational, health, or social work setting, as well as professionals in the field, and parents. It is targeted for people who work or plan to work with children from pre-school to high school and will be useful to teachers, youth leaders, coaches, counselors, social workers, and nurses.

David A. Bergin teaches in the teacher education and graduate programs at the University of Missouri, USA. Dr. Bergin holds PhD and Educational Specialist degrees from Stanford University and has studied topics such as classroom engagement, interest, and motivation for learning. His co-authored textbook for teachers has been used by thousands of students.

Applying Child and Adolescent Development in the Professions Series

Dr. Kimberly A. Gordon Biddle
Series Editor

The field of Child and Adolescent Development is being recognized and legitimized more and more as good preparation for a variety of careers in various fields such as; psychology, education, allied health, non-profits, and social work. As more theories are created and research is conducted, more attention and recognition is given to the field of Child and Adolescent Development.

This series takes core and current topics in the field of Child and Adolescent Development, defines the topics, describes the topics as they develop in children from infancy to age 25 or describes how the topic impacts children from infancy to age 25, and then applies them to careers in five main fields, psychology, education, allied health, non-profits, and social work. Various application strategies and techniques are shared. The core topics addressed in this series of books are as follows; attachment, motivation, social and emotional competence, executive function, and MultiLingual and MultiCultural Development. The current niche topics represented in the series are these; transformative frames for anti-racism, socio-cultural deprivation, and growth mindset for transformative thinking. The writing level is accessible and engaging for students in high school and the first or second year of college. However, the information may be useful for graduate students, too. These books are excellent for early, mid, and late career professionals, too. Employee training and professional development can be enriched with the books of this series.

It is the intention of the book authors that the volumes are helpful to all people who work with and care for children. Indeed, the topics explored in Applying Child and Adolescent Development in the Professions Series move the field forward.

Dr. Kimberly A. Gordon Biddle spent 30 years working full-time in the field of Child and Adolescent Development, with 2 years as a Research Analyst and 28 years as a College Professor. Currently, she is an Emeritus Professor of Child and Adolescent Development from Sacramento State in California. Her BA is in Psychology and Music from the University of Redlands. Her EdS is in Program Evaluation and her PhD is in Child and Adolescent Development. Both of her advanced degrees are from Stanford University.

Over her career she has been an American Psychological Association MFP fellow. She has authored or co-authored over 20 articles and some book chapters. She has presented or co-presented over 40 presentations. Before being the overall editor of this series she had co-authored or co-edited 3 textbooks. She has obtained approximately $1,000,000 in grants. Her research and teaching areas of expertise include motivation, academic resilience, social and emotional development, and the education and socialization of marginalized groups. She also has some expertise in field work placement and coordination and policies concerning children and families. Her career efforts have been rewarded. For example, she has received Outstanding Teaching and Service Awards from Sacramento State. She also won a Stanford Graduate School of Education Award for Excellence in Education in 2018 and a Career Award from the University of Redlands in 2019.

She is thrilled that Routledge asked her to be the lead editor of this book series and she has enjoyed nurturing the series into life. This series is near and dear to her heart and she is honored to edit it and co-author two of the books. She firmly believes that this book series will move the field of Child and Adolescent Development forward. Core concepts of the field and current topics of the field are explored and applied in an engaging manner. Dr. Biddle firmly believes that knowledge of the field of Child and Adolescent Development can assist so many people, whether they are family members of children or are in careers working with children. This series aims to assist those in a wide range of careers who work with children. Those aims are met and surpassed in this series in the opinion of Dr. Biddle. It is her hope that this series is used with students in secondary, undergraduate, and graduate education settings in addition to adults in the fields of education, psychology, social work, allied health, and non-profit organizations. This series is the jewel in Dr. Biddle's career crown. She hopes it shines brightly.

Inspiring Motivation in Children and Youth
How to Nurture Environments for Learning
By David A. Bergin

Inspiring Motivation in Children and Youth

How to Nurture Environments for Learning

David A. Bergin

Routledge
Taylor & Francis Group

NEW YORK AND LONDON

First published 2023
by Routledge
605 Third Avenue, New York, NY 10158

and by Routledge
4 Park Square, Milton Park, Abingdon, Oxon OX14 4RN

Routledge is an imprint of the Taylor & Francis Group, an informa business

Library of Congress Cataloging-in-Publication Data
A catalog record for this title has been requested

ISBN: 978-0-367-49540-4 (hbk)
ISBN: 978-0-367-49541-1 (pbk)
ISBN: 978-1-003-04651-6 (ebk)

DOI: 10.4324/9781003046516

Typeset in Times New Roman
by Taylor & Francis Books

Contents

Acknowledgements

I thank the following for providing comments, feedback, and vignettes: Allison Kerr, Delaney Jackson, Jacala Hartman, Zachery Hackbarth, Amanda Engelke, Molly Finnegan, Kirsten Pinto, Kevin Pugh, Michelle Oliver, Chris Holmes, Leigh Maddy, Jerry Lynn Crosby.

Series Editor Foreward

The field of Child and Adolescent Development is in infant stages of development, but it is steadily maturing. It is time for it be recognized and legitimized. As the theorizing and conduction of research in the field become more solid, complex, and applicable to life, recognition comes that the field is for people in a variety of professions. The traditional education and psychology fields are enriched with the knowledge obtained from the field of Child and Adolescent Development. Additionally, allied health, social work, and non-profit fields are improved with knowledge of how to apply Child and Adolescent Development in the workplace setting. Everyone who works with or cares for children from birth to 25 years will benefit from reading and applying the information from the books in this series. Collectively, the authors have created books rich with foundational information and application techniques and strategies. Thematic boxes of interviews, case studies, and research and theory into practice run throughout all the books. These books help to answer some of the most important questions concerning children and their development. All who love and care about children should read every book in the series.

Dr. Bergin's book on motivation is a true hallmark creation. It defines what it really means to be learned and how to help children and adolescents along the path. The goals, feelings of efficacy, feelings of belonging, and feelings of autonomy that enrich motivation are all described. Additionally, useful strategies and techniques for motivating children and adolescents are shared and described in detail. This book also relays topics such as the influence of competition on motivation, how membership in marginalized communities impacts motivation, and more tips for applying motivational principles in specific workplace settings. Motivating children and adolescents to create adaptive behavior is a question asked continually by professionals and everyday people. This book shares how to do just that in a manner that is engaging and approachable.

Dr. Kimberly A. Gordon Biddle

Introduction

This is a book about motivation in children and youth; it is about how to inspire them to learn and want to change behavior. It is targeted for anyone who works with youth. That includes teachers, parents, coaches, social workers, psychologists, athletic trainers, physical therapists, dieticians, speech language pathologists, health educators, and others. Some sections of the book will be more relevant to one group than to others.

The book is about how to create motivating environments. Many people have erroneous beliefs about motivation. One is that people either have or don't have motivation. When you believe this, you are not inclined to adjust the environment to support motivation.

The other erroneous belief is that you can force people to become motivated. You cannot force people to do your bidding. There is always a dance of influence between the teacher and the learner. The teacher can create environments that inspire motivation and can invite learners to participate in learning activities. The learner can accept or reject these invitations. More enticing invitations are more likely to be successful. Invitations that are attractive can vary by cultural background, gender, religion, individual interests, and other personal and group attributes.

All of the stories in this book are true.

The interviews were mostly conducted by posing written questions to professionals and asking them to write a response.

I have written this book with teachers and health professionals in mind along with those who hope to work in these professions. While you may see "students" or "learners" mentioned in one place and "client" mentioned somewhere else, in reality, I am talking about all of the children and youth with whom you may work.

There is no good single word that encompasses the age group that is targeted by this book. The term "child" can refer to a person between birth and puberty. It can also refer to a person who has not reached full maturity or legal age. The term "youth" can refer to a person between childhood and maturity or a person in adolescence or young adulthood.

This book is targeted for birth to young adulthood, especially persons of school age, so "children and youth" fits but is wordy. Therefore, the text will sometimes refer to children *or* youth but means to include both, and it will also use the term "learners" to refer to children and youth.

Chapter 1

Why is it Important to be a Learned Person?

Part of the role of adults who teach or influence children and youth is to help them become learned. This requires fostering curiosity and motivation to learn. It is hard to imagine a scenario in which our children would be better off if they learned less. In fact, their lives will be better in terms of enjoyment, health, and income if they learn more. Teachers, parents, coaches, physical therapists, dieticians, speech language pathologists, dental hygienists and others who work with and teach children and youth want them to become learned because learning influences their well-being and their probability of following therapeutic guidance.

This book takes the stance that people who educate should help motivate children and youth to become "learned." By learned, I mean

- Broad background knowledge
- Critical thinking skills
- Problem solving skills
- Curiosity to continue learning new things

A person does not really "become" learned, as though it is a destination where you can arrive and be finished with the journey. Becoming learned is a process that continues.

Our national and global communities would be better off if children, at a young age, were motivated to understand current events, health information, literature, popular culture, geography, mathematics, and many other topics. They would not ask "will it be on the test?" They would want to know to satisfy their own curiosity and so that they can contribute as knowledgeable citizens. For example, in order to understand global politics, people need to know where Pakistan is geographically in relation to India and Afghanistan. In order to write reports to bosses and recommendation letters for students, adults must be able to write letters and emails that are coherent and convincing. Such global knowledge and writing competence are not skills that you pick up on the spur of the moment; they come from motivation to learn.

DOI: 10.4324/9781003046516-1

A learned person would be motivated to have some understanding of mathematics. Americans tend to be averse to math, but often unexpectedly find that they need to understand math. For example, they may read a news story that Black students are disproportionately given more severe punishment than White students for the same misbehavior. What does disproportionate mean in that context? According to data from the Department of Education, Black students made up 18% of those enrolled in the K-12 schools sampled, but they accounted for 35% of those suspended once, 46% of those suspended more than once, and 39% of all expulsions (Lewin, 2012). One can see that if a group is 18% of the sample and 35% of those suspended, the group is suspended at a higher rate—disproportionate—than other racial-ethnic groups.

A learned person would understand that sun exposure is linked with skin cancer, that dental hygiene is linked with tooth decay, and calorie-dense foods are linked with obesity. But not everyone knows these things. And even those who do know don't necessarily act on their knowledge, which brings us to the topic of inert knowledge.

Inert Knowledge

A problem with knowledge is that it can be inert. That is, a person can have knowledge but not be motivated to draw upon it or not know how to draw upon it. Alfred Whitehead, English mathematician and philosopher, wrote,

> we must be aware of what I will call 'inert ideas'—that is to say, ideas that are merely received into the mind without being utilized, or tested, or thrown into fresh combination.... Education with inert ideas is not only useless: it is, above all things, harmful.
> (Whitehead, 1959, reprinted from 1929, p. 193)

People can know about behaviors that decrease the probability of disease and the benefits of investing while young but not use the knowledge.

An example of inert knowledge comes from mathematics. In what is now a famous task (Reusser, 1988), 97 first and second graders were presented the problem, "There are 26 sheep and 10 goats on a ship. How old is the captain?" (pp. 324–325). Seventy-six of the students "solved" the task with "36."

The same author reported the following problem and response:

> There are 125 sheep and 5 dogs in a flock. How old is the shepherd?" One student responded: "125+5=130 ... this is too big, and 125–5=120 is still too big ... while ... 125/5=25 ... that works ... I think the shepherd is 25 years old."
> (p. 325)

In this case, the student engaged in logical thinking and recognized that 130 and 120 are too old for a shepherd, but was not logical enough to recognize that the problem makes no sense. The student saw a school-type of problem and proceeded to solve. The student was not yet learned.

In another example, 5th and 6th graders were presented the following problem (Renkl et al., 1996, p 117):

> The 130 students and teachers from Marie Curie School are going on a picnic. Each school bus holds 50 passengers. How many buses will they need?
> a) 2; b) 2 R30; c) 2 3/5; d) 3.

Many students chose b or c. It did not occur to them that you cannot have fractions of a bus. Part of being learned is not being seduced into nonsense problem solving.

Reusser (1988) described a physics student who gave the "correct" school-based answer and then had some fun. In a physics exam, the student was asked,

> Show how one can measure the height of a skyscraper with the help of a barometer

The student gave the correct answer: "One can determine the height of the building by reading off from the barometer the air pressure difference between road and roof. Air pressure decreases by 1 Torr (=1mm Hg) approximately every 30 feet" (p. 321). The student then teased the reader with six added responses. I present three of them:

a   You take the barometer with you to the top of the roof, tie it to a long rope and lower it to the road. Then you pull it back up and measure the length of the rope. This length corresponds to the height of the skyscraper.

b   You take the barometer to the top of the building. Then you lean out over the edge of the roof. You drop the barometer and measure the falling time with a stopwatch. Then you determine the height of the building by the law of falling bodies: $d = \frac{1}{2} gt^2$.

c   Finally, if you do not want me to commit myself to a physics solution, then there still are many more possibilities. For example, you could take the barometer and knock on the caretaker's door. If he answers the door, then you speak as follows: "Dear caretaker, I have here an exciting barometer. If you tell me the height of the building, then it's yours." (pp. 320–321)

This student understood the task, answered it, and then showed creativity and wit. That seems like someone who is becoming learned.

What is Learning?

Becoming learned requires learning, of course. Three long-time professors of learning came to an agreement, apparently after considerable discussion and disagreement, about the principles that are foundational to understanding human learning (Alexander et al., 2009). I will comment on five of the principles. First, *Learning is change*. As we learn, we change. That change can come in physical abilities like being able to skip, hit a pitched ball, or run faster. That change can also come in our cognitive abilities to speak a language, solve problems, or teach others. Later in this book, I will discuss transformative experience, which refers to learning that changes how we see and experience the world. Will a person who has seen the film *Super Size Me*, about a guy who for one month ate all his meals at McDonalds and suffered negative health consequences as a result, including puking, ever see fast food with the same eyes? When we learn new things, we see our environment with different eyes. A goal of people who work with children and youth should be that the young people be motivated to use the new knowledge in their lives. Why teach music if learners do not change how they create or appreciate music? Why teach literature if learners do not change how they read and understand books? Why teach physical therapy exercises if the learners don't use them? Why coach sports if young athletes do not learn teamwork and healthy habits?

Principle 2 is that *Learning is inevitable, essential, and constant*. Everyone learns as a result of functioning in the world. Children learn language. They don't set out to learn language. They don't ask for lessons. They just learn their native language. Children in schools learn social skills as a result of interacting with other kids. They don't say to themselves, "I need to learn how to join a group of agemates who are conversing." Everyone in their sphere engages socially, so they learn too.

The third principle is *Learning can be resisted*. People sometimes resist learning, like British working-class "lads" who rejected schooling because they felt no motivation to go along with school expectations that would not bring upward mobility and were not worth the effort (McGrew, 2011). Many schools have students who resist learning and trying to get good grades because they are afraid of criticism from peers (Bishop et al., 2004). Learners may resist learning because it is difficult.

The fourth principle is *Learning can be disadvantageous*. Students can learn to disrupt or divert their teacher, perhaps by talking about a recent sports event or asking what the teacher will do during an upcoming holiday. Such a strategy is advantageous for avoiding work, but is disadvantageous in the long term because it undermines learning. Learning can also be disadvantageous when children and youth learn bad habits like smoking and drinking that threaten their health. They can learn aggression, which gets them things in the short term, but undermines their social competence and circle of friends in the long run.

The fifth principle is *Learning can be tacit and incidental as well as conscious and intentional*. Everyone picks up information incidentally as well as intentionally, but the learned person is more intentional about their incidental learning. They notice that on the New York subway, you don't sit next to someone on an empty subway car. They remember the name of the president of Mexico. The learned person is alert to information that they did not intentionally seek but that fills in their personal web of knowledge.

Learning Supports Comprehension

Motivation to become learned is important for comprehension and understanding. People who have broad knowledge more easily understand what they read and observe than people with more restricted knowledge. One key reading skill is the ability to decode words, that is, to be able to say the word or recognize the word. But just because you can decode "infamous" does not mean that you understand it. Many people think it is a variant of "famous" when it really means well-known for bad or evil behavior, which can lead to all sorts of misconceptions for people who lack relevant knowledge.

If you are reading a story that takes place in Europe in August 1939, what should you anticipate in the story? It is nearly inevitable that the story will include the start of WW2 in Europe on September 1, 1939. One person might have no clue what was coming, another might anticipate WW2, and a third might understand nuances of 1939 politics in France, Germany, and Poland. Who has greater comprehension? The same principles apply to movies and conversations.

A child might be able to decode words like *shell, sand*, and *beach*, but without understanding what the words mean will make little sense of a beach story. Consider a story with words like *love, ad one, 40, game*, and *set*. Or a story that refers to *basting, bias, bobbin*, and *frogging*. People who understand the contexts of tennis and sewing are much more likely to understand and enjoy the stories or discussions than those who do not.

Consider the following passages from popular books:

- *Anne of Green Gables* refers to "bearding a lion in its den" (p. 19), a carpetbag, an orphan in an asylum (p. 21), a buggy, and a wincey dress (three hundred yards of wincey, p. 23).
- *Stuart Little* refers to a sticky piano key (p. 7), a louse instead of a mouse (p.10), and a mouse rolling up in a shade (p. 19).
- *Harry Potter and the Chamber of Secret*, refers to crack like a whip (p.19), cat-flap (p. 22), pick the lock (p. 26), and load of dung (p. 29).

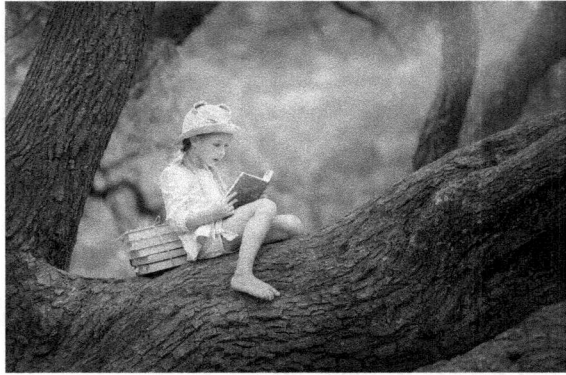

You can imagine the misconceptions that young readers might have about a buggy, sticky keys, a mouse in a shade, and crack like a whip; misconceptions could undermine motivation to read.

Similar problems can arise for late adolescents who read non-fiction. For example, the first two pages of the Pulitzer Prize winning book *The Looming Tower* refer to a cell of Islamic terrorists, electronic ears, fight the Cold War, jaded king, fatwa, and neck-smiting. What might a young person who did not live through the Cold War or read John le Carré novels make of such phrases? A person who is becoming learned builds up the background knowledge to understand such vocabulary and looks up or asks about at least some unfamiliar words and phrases.

A study of background knowledge found that there is a threshold effect; that is, below a certain amount of knowledge, there is little relationship between knowledge and reading comprehension (O'Reilly et al., 2019). Above the threshold, the more a reader knows, the better their comprehension. The study also showed that vocabulary is crucial for reading comprehension, and the bigger the vocabulary, the better the comprehension. There is a push to emphasize academic vocabulary because of similar research findings (e.g., Bae et al., 2021). For example, in science education, learners must understand science vocabulary to understand the science. In geology, vocabulary includes words for eras (e.g., mesozoic and paleozoic), minerals (e.g., quartz and calcite), and rocks (igneous, sedimentary, and metamorphic). Each area of science has distinct vocabulary.

Responsible Citizens

Motivation to understand science is part of becoming learned and responsible citizens. There seems to be increasing science denial, which can be defined as rejecting empirical evidence to avoid undesirable facts or conclusions (Darner, 2019) or as using arguments that give the appearance of legitimate debate where there is none because a scientific consensus already exists based on data (Diethelm & McKee, 2009). The learned person understands that science is based on the scientific method, and its conclusions can change based on new data; nevertheless, scientific consensus gives the best estimate of current knowledge. Science denial has cost tens of thousands of lives because some people did not believe the scientific consensus about what causes AIDS, whether smoking causes illness, or whether seat belts protect lives. The learned person accepts science with its flaws and rejects reasoning that relies on selectivity, misrepresentation, and logical fallacies.

Using the internet is part of becoming learned and responsible citizens. Knowing where to turn for information is important and influences voting, medical decisions, and consumer decisions. Many people lack motivation to discover the sources of internet information. For example, a nice website that looks professional and displays misleading data in graphs and charts can deceive even knowledgeable people. To assess the accuracy of a website, you must look outside of the website.

A group of researchers at Stanford (Breakstone et al., 2021) found that even college professors tended to look inside of a website for evidence of reliability (who claims to run it, what is their stated goal, what are the quality of the graphics, do they cite data, etc.) instead of looking outside of the website to see what other experts say about reliability. They called looking outside "lateral reading" (looking outside of a website for clues about reliability such as who funds it) instead of "vertical reading" (reading a website from top to bottom looking for clues inside of the website). The Stanford researchers gave high school students six tasks that involved assessing accuracy of online information. For example, in the Website Evaluation Task, students were given a link to a website and asked if it was a "reliable source for information about global warming." They found that students were dismally bad at assessing the website, which was funded by fossil fuel companies; 96.8% received the lowest score. One student wrote, "This page is a reliable source to obtain information from. You see in the URL that it ends in .org as opposed to .com" (p. 509). The student apparently did not know that .org is an "open" domain, which means that anyone can obtain it.

On the Evaluating Evidence Task, students were presented a link to a video of ballot stuffing supposedly in the United States. Of the 3119 responses on that task, only three students tracked down the source of the video, which was from a Russian election, not a US election. Out of 3,446 students, at least two thirds used incorrect or irrelevant strategies for each of the six tasks. Results from this study and others show that American teens, and college professors, are poorly prepared for assessing the reliability of information on internet websites; nevertheless, with motivation and guidance, they can improve.

Intrinsic Motivation

As people pursue becoming learned, they are likely to feel intrinsic motivation for learning new things. Intrinsic motivation refers to the desire to pursue an activity for its own sake, not for external reasons. In contrast, extrinsic motivation refers to engaging in an activity for external reasons, that is, because it is instrumental to achieving something outside the activity—like getting a job, earning money, getting praise from others, pleasing parents, or impressing friends. Experiencing intrinsic motivation for all of your activities is impossible. It is not likely that children and youth you know engage in classroom learning activities because they find every activity interesting and desirable. This is also true of athletes and clients. Learners you work with are likely to feel a mix of intrinsic and extrinsic motivation.

People often confuse intrinsic motivation with the desire to do an activity. That is not accurate. A student could desire to take a required course in order to fulfill requirements, which is extrinsic motivation. An athlete could want to practice in order to become a better athlete, also extrinsic. Intrinsic motivation only occurs when the person likes to do the activity for its own sake. Students in school seldom feel intrinsic motivation for school tasks because they would not choose to do those tasks if they could do anything that they wanted. For example, they might be intrinsically motivated to read books that they choose, but they are seldom intrinsically motivated to read books assigned in school or to write the required book reports and papers. They might be intrinsically motivated to play a sport, but they are seldom intrinsically motivated to do physical therapy recommended by a therapist. The topic of intrinsic motivation will be discussed further in Chapter 4.

A Preference for Challenge

Children and youth who want to become learned prefer challenge. Mathematics is challenging for many children and youth, and in the US, they tend to avoid difficult mathematics. A study asked over 7,000 ninth graders if they would rather do an extra credit math assignment that would be easy but with little learning or a challenging task that would be difficult and would foster new learning; 63% chose the easy task (Rege et al., 2021). One line of research that has investigated preference for challenge examined whether people believe that their ability is changeable and can grow—growth mindset—or believe that their ability is fixed and unchangeable—fixed mindset. When children and youth believe that their ability is fixed, they tend to avoid challenges. A set of studies in the US and Norway (Rege et al., 2021) found that after an intervention that taught a growth mindset, students were more likely to prefer challenging math problems and to enroll in advanced math classes. They were more interested in becoming learned. However, the intervention only worked in schools that made it easy to move up to challenging classes. Thus, the intervention requires a change in the person *and* a responsive environment. Mindset is discussed more in Chapter 2.

On the Path to Becoming Learned

Individuals who are motivated to become learned want to understand the world and their place in it. Consider student William Martin, who had various learning disabilities as a child and struggled in school, but as a teen loved to learn about the Civil War (Neu et al., 2004). He was intensely interested in learning new things. William heard that during the Civil War, at the Battle of Shiloh, some soldiers' wounds seemed to glow, and those soldiers seemed to have a lower death rate. William and his friend decided to do a science fair project to see if it was possible that bacteria caused the glowing *and* the reduced death rate. They found that certain bacteria that likely existed at Shiloh do glow and do create antibiotics that inhibit the growth of harmful bacteria. With their research, they won the Intel ISEF Competition.

Eliza McNitt got stuck in a high school hands-on research class because it was the only science class that fit her schedule (Dutton, 2011). She was no science nerd and was not really interested in the course, but she had to think of a project. She wondered about pesticides on apples, which made her think about foods that could not easily be cleaned of pesticides, which made her wonder if honey contains pesticides. That led to finding that honey does contain pesticides, and she placed second in the Environmental Management category in the Intel Science and Engineering Fair. The next year she and a classmate won a C-SPAN documentary film competition with their *Requiem for the Honeybee,* and her research on Colony Collapse Disorder won Best in Category at the Intel ISEF. She and her fellow science fair participants were learning to be learned.

The perceived value of learning can increase in situations of deprivation. A former POW in Vietnam wrote of his time in a prisoner of war camp in North Vietnam (Chesley, 1973),

> Our hunger for knowledge was almost as great as our hunger for food—in some respects, perhaps even greater. How different it might have been if I had had just one good book—preferably the scriptures, but even Shakespeare or a dictionary, for example! In prison, we were so hungry for reading material that the labels on our occasional packages from home (before the authorities started taking them from us) were probably a greater joy to us even than eating the goodies. We spent hours studying those labels—reading the instructions, spelling out the ingredients, calculating the weights from listed details, and

reveling in every way in the delights of this printed word. My hunger
for knowledge was stimulated by the deprivation, of course. It was not
always there previously. As with most young people, I suppose, I had
gone to college not with a yearning for true education but with the
goal of getting out of college as fast as I could, of getting the grades
and the diploma. I achieved that goal without learning much then
promptly forgot what I *had* learned.

(p. 74)

Imagine having students who felt that motivated to read and learn. The
former POW went on to list the lessons that the POW's gave each other on
American history, psychology, religion, French, Spanish, German, and
trigonometry. The greatest interest was in American history and second in
religion. They memorized poems and Bible verses. They even had music
lessons without instruments and dance lessons without music.

I end this chapter with the story of Ryan Green (Bergner, 2016), who
struggled to become learned. Because of difficult life circumstances, much
of his life was a struggle, but once he got the vision of learning and artistic
expression, he was motivated to continually learn and improve. He found
motivation within, and was also supported by teachers and institutions:

> Ryan Green, who is Black, grew up observing domestic violence from
> his mother, father, and step-father. His mother was once knocked
> unconscious by his step-father. His brother went to prison. Ryan was
> kicked out of four preschool day care centers for violent and dis-
> ruptive behavior. An elementary school principal said, "He was one of
> the ten or so most troubled children I've had in my forty-two-year
> career. I recall his teacher actually taking all the other children out of
> the room in order to protect them" (Bergner, 2016, pp. 46–47). His
> teacher, Mrs. Hughes, was dedicated to improving the lives of her
> students. She selected books for them, had them memorize lines from
> Martin Luther King's "I have a dream" speech, and devised special
> lessons for each. When Ryan was in sixth grade, he attacked his
> mother with a knife. Authorities locked him up in a center for trou-
> bled youth. He played Nintendo, called other kids jackasses, threa-
> tened to kill a girl, and threatened to rip the f—ing faces off of staff.
> He was big for his age and threatening. Mrs. Hughes phoned and
> tried to reassure him. He was finally released to live with his mother.
> He went to school. He tried to learn formal English by imitating the
> speech patterns of the *ER* television show and of television news
> anchors. He wanted to learn new things, joined the Latin club, read
> *The Cat in the Hat* in Latin, and participated in Latin quiz bowls.
> Ryan was on the eighth-grade football team. The coach encouraged
> him to take chorus for an easy credit, and the chorus teacher pushed

the students to audition for the Governor's School for the Arts, a pull-out program for half of each school day. It turned out the principal of the Governor's school was the husband of Mrs. Hughes. Out of all the arts, Ryan tried out for opera. The opera program needed boys, so despite his mediocre tryout, he was accepted for his freshman year. He started making the honor roll in school and was accused of acting white. At Governor's, he was trying to learn to read music, understand classical music, and sing as his voice was changing. This was a tremendous learning load. His sophomore year, he was taught by Mr. Brown, an African American educator who took Ryan under his wing. That year, Ryan went on a school trip to the Metropolitan Opera in New York City. Ryan loved the production of *Carmen* and announced, "I'm going to sing at the Met" (Bergner, 2016, p. 153). Mr. Brown continued to work with Ryan, helped clothe him, and gave him driving lessons. Ryan's singing skills improved. He went to college and studied music on scholarship. He competed in the Met's opera competition and was one of five winners. He was admitted to the Met's developmental program, where he struggled because he lacked the background knowledge and experience of other performers. Despite his struggles, he continued to improve. After overcoming many challenges, Ryan did perform at the Met as a professional opera singer.

While few people will face the challenges that Ryan Green faced, everyone will face challenges. Teachers, therapists, and coaches can help learners develop motivational resources that provide the energy to overcome challenges. Ryan Green's experiences illustrate topics that will be discussed in this book such as goals, belongingness, background knowledge, and ethnic-racial influences. His experience also illustrates the importance of mentors and advocates.

The Coming Chapters

The book is structured with chapters about five approaches to thinking about motivation: goals; competence; belongingness; autonomy; and making learning meaningful, relevant, and interesting. Then the book discusses two overarching topics that are relevant to motivation: competition and diversity. The final chapter applies motivation concepts to helping professions such as counseling, psychotherapy, social work, and allied health professions.

Summary

- To be learned should be a goal.
- Inert knowledge, that is, knowledge that you are not motivated to use or don't know how to use, is a problem in learning situations.

- Learning

  a is change
  b is inevitable, essential, and constant
  c can be resisted
  d can be disadvantageous
  e can be tacit and incidental as well as conscious and intentional

- Learning supports comprehension and understanding. The more you know, the easier it is to understand text, movies, lectures, conversations, and other situations.
- Responsible citizens attempt to be learned. Assessing information on the internet can be particularly important.
- Intrinsic motivation refers to the desire to pursue an activity for its own sake, not for external reasons. It is often misunderstood.
- People who are motivated to become learned want to understand the world and their place in it.

Suggestions for Further Reading

Brophy, J. (2008). Developing students' appreciation for what is taught in school. *Educational Psychologist, 43*(3), 132–141.

Kohn, Alfie. Online essay on "What does it mean to be well-educated?" www.alfiekohn.org/article/mean-well-educated-article/

Chapter 2

What Goals do Children and Youth Have? How do Goals Influence their Behavior?

A goal is an intention to achieve future valued outcomes. Research consistently shows that goals affect motivation and performance. This has been demonstrated in settings including schools, sports, healthcare, factories, and sales (Locke & Latham, 1990; 2013). There is further discussion of goals in Chapter 9.

How do goals work? Goals direct attention. If I have a goal to improve my relationship with my children, my attention repeatedly focuses on that topic. My attention will be caught by articles and conversations that focus on parenting. I will seek out websites that discuss parent-child relationships.

Goals foster persistence. If I am committed to a goal to earn a master's degree even though I work full time, when I get home from work, I will be more likely to pull out the books and study. As I start to doze off while studying, I am more likely to snap to attention and continue studying.

Goals foster strategies. If I set an explicit goal to improve client outcomes, I am likely to develop improved strategies for providing therapy. I am likely to read books and watch videos on therapy. I am likely to seek feedback, even though it might feel threatening, from expert therapists. When goals direct attention, foster persistence, and foster strategies, they also improve performance.

In the next sections, I will focus on three aspects of goals:

1   where do goals come from
2   what are achievement goals
3   how does one set goals

Where do Goals Come From?

People get their goals from various sources. Let's start with families, a key influence on goals. When children are raised in a family, they receive messages about what kinds of work, sports, and hobbies are suitable for people like them. A study of immigrant Mexican families found that children's career goals tended to follow their parents' aspirations (Behnke

DOI: 10.4324/9781003046516-2

et al., 2004); for example, parents who wanted to become better educated tended to have children who were interested in attending college. Studies of youth sports find that families influence their children to have sports goals (Birchwood et al., 2008; Hayoz et al., 2017; Wheeler, 2011).

Families may influence students' goals in stereotypical ways. For example, studies have shown that parents tend to have higher mathematics expectations for boys than for girls (Gunderson et al., 2012). Parents often believe that their sons have more natural talent in math than their daughters.

Families may also influence goals through communicating gender and ethnic-racial stereotypes about other activities such as which sports are appropriate, should you seek counseling, what careers should you pursue, and so forth. Any family member can communicate beliefs about what goals a child or youth should adopt; influential family members can include parents, grandparents, siblings, aunts, uncles, and cousins.

Parents communicate their goals for their children through the opportunities they provide. For example, parents communicate a goal for musical competence when they provide piano lessons. They give up their own time and money to pay for lessons and transport their children to lessons. Parents sign their children up for Lego robotics, gymnastics, summer coding camp, cheerleading, and so forth. Each activity communicates the goal to become competent in the activity. Parents also communicate goals such as being popular, attractive, athletic, smart, and a winner.

Pushing kids to participate in activities is class-based, with middle-class parents using "concerted cultivation" of their children and working-class parents allowing "natural growth" (Lareau, 2003). Concerted cultivation refers to the middle-class pattern of parents actively fostering their children's talents and skills through lessons in a deliberate attempt to help them get ahead. Natural growth refers to working-class and poor parents' pattern of allowing their children's development to unfold spontaneously. Thus, middle-class parents are more likely to explicitly impose goals on their children. At the same time, they are more likely to assess their children's own goals and then pull together resources to support those goals. For example, if they notice that their child likes to draw, they might buy drawing books and sign the child up for drawing lessons.

Socioeconomic status (SES), which refers to status based on wealth, income, education, and occupational prestige, is a major influence on goals. For children, SES comes from parents. SES influences people's expectations for achieving the goal of getting ahead. It makes sense that people would want to get ahead because getting ahead leads to higher status, better health, and better prospects for one's children (Laurin, 2016). However, not everyone has the goal of higher income with greater status. Individuals from low-income backgrounds may perceive that they cannot overcome systemic barriers, or that they cannot gain access to effective role models and mentoring, or that they do not desire the political maneuvering that comes with higher status jobs (Laurin, 2016). They may want to maintain their existing ethnic, cultural, or social identity and show solidarity with friends and family. One Appalachian woman who cleaned houses in a midwestern city said that

> Her only needs were enough money to pay the bills, buy food to eat, and have enough left over for fun like "four-wheelin'" on the weekends. She felt sorry for some of the women she worked for who shared with her their worries about being robbed or losing their money to greedy relatives. She didn't want the "headaches" that she believed wealth would bring.
>
> (Purcell-Gates, 1995, p. 28)

When thinking about people's motivation, it is important to think about their goals. Are they motivated for a particular career or are they motivated to retain their economic position? High-income children and youth are pushed to have goals for high-status education and careers (Binder & Abel, 2018; Schleef, 2000). When asked why she went to law school after giving up on medicine, one student answered

> I had thought but not seriously about going into nursing, but then I thought that's a big step down from becoming a doctor.... I guess I'm ambitious and I want my family to be proud of me.... A law profession or doctor is very prestigious, and parents like to tell their friends, "My daughter's in law school," so that pushes me, too.
>
> (Schleef, 2000, p. 162)

Was this student motivated to become a doctor or lawyer? Or was she motivated to maintain her level of prestige?

When asked why go to business school, an MBA student said,

> If you looked at my training class, it's almost like growing up in a way, where if you come from certain backgrounds, be it upper class, certain things are expected of you. You're going to get a decent high school education, you're going to go to a very good college, and then maybe you'll go on to get a very good job, maybe you'll pursue graduate [studies].
>
> (Schleef, 2000, p. 166)

These examples show that career goals and motivation often come from socioeconomic background and cultural pressure.

A study of the goal to become a teacher found influences from family, teachers, peers, and previous teaching experiences (Schutz et al., 2001). In addition, emotions played a role, like the teacher who said that when she visited her old school, "I got chills when I walked in the school because I was just like 'This is what I want'" (p. 303).

Cultural background, ethnic-racial group, gender, and SES influence goals such as which sport to play and what kind of music to acquire. In terms of sports, lacrosse tends to be more popular in the US northeast than in other areas. Baseball, which is popular in parts of Latin America like Cuba and Nicaragua, is increasingly popular with Latinx youth in the US. Soccer ("football" outside of the US) is less popular in the US than in other areas of the world. Golf and tennis tend to be sports for white middle- to upper-income athletes.

Music is an important part of ethnic identity. At dances and schoolwide events, Latinx and African American students at one high school argued about the types of music that would be played—salsa and merengue vs rap, house, rhythm and blues, and soul. "African-American students decried the excess of 'Spanish music' at the same time that Latino students bemoaned the prevalence of 'Black music'" (Jacob, 1995, p. 359). Similar conflict occurred in the military. In his autobiography, General Colin Powell reported that there was race friction based on musical preference at bars near a US military camp in Korea.

> "The whites wanted rock and country-and-western. The blacks wanted soul, Aretha Franklin, and Dionne Warwick.... They finally agreed that they would feature roughly seven 'white' songs for every three 'black' songs. As a result of the compromise, the whites were unhappy only 30 percent of the time and the blacks 70 percent"
>
> (Powell, 1995, p. 189).

Cultural stereotypes can influence goals. For example, stereotypes that girls and youth of color have low competence in STEM domains (science, technology, engineering, mathematics) can undermine their STEM goals. Such stereotypes may help explain why there are fewer women and students of color in STEM fields.

Some research has investigated goal contagion in which people "catch" their friends' and colleagues' goals (Laurin, 2016). This pattern influences parents to buy homes in certain neighborhoods and to create sport and hobby opportunities for their children. The youth in the surrounding neighborhood, sports teams, and hobby lessons serve as models. Parents believe that their children catch goals from peers; that is why they buy homes that are served by certain schools and why some parents put their children in private schools. They want their children exposed to some goals and deprived of exposure to other goals. Parents cannot completely control goal exposure, but they can influence it.

Teachers directly influence goals by modeling goals themselves, inviting guest speakers who model goals, and suggesting goals. Therapists directly influence goals by suggesting them or by collaborating with a client to develop a set of goals (Rohde et al., 2012). Coaches directly influence goals by helping teams and individuals set goals (Weinberg, 2010).

Interview: Goals

Elementary Teacher at a Suburban School. Two Years of Experience

I found the idea that parents influence goals to be really interesting for both professional and personal reasons. Both of my parents were D1 athletes and put me in sports when I was nine months old. They always had high expectations for me in sports, and it wasn't about "fun" but about winning. Now, even as an adult, I find I really struggle to accept doing anything if I'm not the best and have the mindset that if I'm going to do something, I need to be the best at it. I recently picked up roller skating just for a fun activity, and I realized it's the first time I've ever done an activity solely because I enjoy it and not because I want to win. Their expectations for me set me up for how I think for years to come. I've also seen this in my students so far this year, so that if their parents don't have high expectations for them, they tend to not have high expectations for themselves.

I also found the familial aspect of goals applied to teaching to be interesting. The majority of teachers I know come from a family of teachers. My grandma and mom were both teachers, and I followed in their footsteps. The principal of the school I work at now has a daughter who teaches in the district. My best friend from undergraduate is a 2nd grade teacher, and her mom is a 5th grade teacher. When I was in undergraduate, when we had to say what inspired us to become teachers, a lot of the answers were "My mom was a teacher, so it was just natural."

Achievement Goals

Learners tend to orient toward two major types of goals in situations where they want to achieve competence: 1) mastery goals, or learning in order to gain understanding, and 2) performance goals, or learning in order to perform better than others, to show others that you are capable, and to avoid looking less capable (Anderman & Wolters, 2006). You can see this in action in youth. When they are in physical therapy, are they focused on improving mobility, or are they monitoring who else is in the gym and wondering who is looking at them and judging them? When they are in a classroom and the teacher asks a question, are they focused on figuring out the answer or on avoiding looking foolish in front of the class? Thus, performance goals involve the ego in ways that mastery goals do not. It is easy to see that anxiety is more likely to be linked with performance goals than with mastery goals

Note that young children are less aware of how they compare to other kids. If you have worked with preschoolers and preadolescents, you may have been surprised when they announced that they were one of the best at a sport or task when in fact they were not; their ability to self-assess and compare to others is poor but improves as they grow.

Case 2.1

A university offers various week-long summer camps. Teens live in the dorms and participate in instruction all day every day. Let's say you invite your teen child to go to soccer summer camp with her soccer all-star cousin even though your daughter does not play soccer competitively. What would your daughter say? Would she focus on learning new skills (mastery goal) or looking stupid (performance goal)? [This dilemma faced a teen I know. She immediately rejected the offer because she thought she would look bad. The parents convinced her that she would not see the other girls again and she would have fun and learn new things. She went and had a good experience. Girls at the camp said she was gutsy and no way would they go to a camp where they would not look good.]

Situations that activate achievement goals are broad. For example, students doing lab experiments may be focused on how they are doing compared to others (performance goal) more than on learning the science concepts (mastery goal). Youth who are meeting new peers for the first time may be concerned about looking socially competent (performance goal) more than on getting to know peers (mastery goal). Learners in physical therapy might be motivated to do easy exercises in order to look good in the gym (performance goals) more than on doing difficult exercises that most aid recovery (mastery goals). In each case, both goals can be highly motivating, but for qualitatively different reasons. This is a key distinction. Both groups can be equally motivated, but for different outcomes.

These two major goals can be divided so that there is an approach and an avoidance dimension of each, resulting in four achievement goals: mastery approach, mastery avoidance, performance approach, and performance avoidance. Mastery avoidance goals have less research support than the others, so I focus on the three-goal model. A *mastery approach* goal refers to striving to learn and master material. A *performance approach* goal refers to striving to demonstrate ability and to do better than others. A *performance avoidance* goal refers to striving to avoid appearing unable and doing worse than others.

Learners tend to think differently about how to engage a task depending on which of these three types of goals they hold. A learner holding a mastery approach goal may want to try difficult tasks, keep going in the face of difficulty, and develop new strategies for success. A learner holding a performance approach goal may also develop strategies for success, but may prefer easier tasks and worry about appearance compared to others. A learner holding a performance avoidance goal is likely to experience anxiety and avoid tasks that look like they might result in failure. In terms of academic achievement like grades, research shows that performance approach goals are related most consistently with success, and mastery goals are also related with high achievement, but less consistently.

However, grades are not the only way to think about success. Mastery goals are also linked with deep learning strategies, intrinsic motivation, growth mindset, and low anxiety. It seems more adaptive for teachers, therapists, and coaches to emphasize mastery goals most of the time, especially during practice, studying, and training. If learners have performance goals and are worried about how they will do in the future, they may experience anxiety that takes up their thinking space and interferes with learning. On the other hand, trying to look smart and to do better than others can be useful during a competition or performance.

For most situations, mastery approach goals should be emphasized over other achievement goals because mastery goals are linked with deeper learning strategies and more positive emotional outcomes like low anxiety. The types of achievement goals a learner shoots for may be the result of relatively stable individual differences (traits) or due to situational influences (states). Instructors and therapists cannot do much to influence stable traits, but they can often arrange situational influences that influence learners' achievement goals toward mastery or performance, approach or avoidance. The following are guidelines that foster mastery approach goals:

- *Provide interesting tasks.* Learners are more likely to engage in efforts to master the content when they think that learning tasks are interesting and meaningful (Bergin, 1999, 2016; Renninger & Hidi, 2011; Turner et al., 2011).
- *Recognize effort and self-improvement.* Recognize and comment on learners' persistence, diligence, and strategy use. Praise learners when they improve. Comment on learners' hard work.
- *Avoid social comparison that pits learners against each other* (Dweck, 1986). Instructors should emphasize learning new skills and trying hard (mastery goals) rather than who is doing the best (competitive goals). Do not publicly display learner's scores or compare learners ("Llami is our most productive student" or "Jack is better at math than Carlos"). Avoiding comparisons also supports a growth mindset, discussed next.
- *Promote a growth mindset* (Dweck & Yeager, 2019). Beliefs about abilities are linked with achievement goals (Dweck, 1986). People who have a fixed mindset – they believe that ability is relatively fixed and

unchangeable – tend to adopt performance goals and thoughts like "*I am not good at math and that will never change.*" They are highly sensitive to comparison with others and the possibility of negative judgments about their ability. They fear failure and see setbacks as threatening. In contrast, people who have a growth mindset – believe that ability can be developed through effort, time, and effective strategies – tend to adopt mastery goals and experience thoughts like "*I am not good at math, but if I practice I will get good at it.*" They like challenges and have less fear of failure because they believe that they learn from failure. As an instructor or therapist, you can influence mindsets (Blackwell et al., 2007; Paunesku et al., 2015), but not easily because learners have spent many years confirming their beliefs that they are good at some things and bad at other things. Think about your own math ability, athletic ability, or art ability. Do you think of yourself as good in some and hopeless in others? Do you have a fixed or growth mindset for your professional skills? To foster a growth mindset, you can teach learners that learning changes the brain by forming new connections and that effort over time with good strategies can improve skills. When clients or students say that they cannot do something or do not like an activity, you can say, "not yet!" (Dweck, 2010). (A mindset intervention is available at no cost to schools at www.perts.net.)

Goal Setting

If children or youth you work with have focused, specific outcomes that they want to achieve, goal setting techniques can be very useful. Many years of research show that goal setting consistently improves performance in just about any domain (Hattie, 2009; Locke & Latham, 2002, 2006; Morisano, 2013). In educational contexts, goals can be broad like achieving high grades or specific like completing a high-quality research project. They can even be specific to an assignment like including at least three pieces of evidence to support each assertion in an essay.

Goals are important in therapeutic areas like physical therapy, occupational therapy, and counseling. The therapist may help the client set specific goals, write them down, and then monitor them. The goals can range from how to improve self-confidence to how many repetitions of an exercise to complete. For example, a White 14-year-old elite hydroplane boat racer and active lacrosse player broke his knee (VanEtten et al., 2021). It was a challenging case because he had poor previous experience with physical therapy, and the surgery outcome was less than ideal. The physical therapist helped set specific objective goals that were based on the demands of hydroplane boat racing. Goals included improving range of motion, strength, and gait. The youth was able to return to racing. The therapist followed up via email five years later. The young man wrote,

Lacrosse and racing the past couple years has been so much fun and I couldn't thank you enough.... You helped me return to that racing season in the summer of 2015 to win my first national championship. Now the crazy part here is after that I have gone on to win six more national championships.

(p. 546)

Research has identified aspects of goal setting that make goals more, or less, effective. Namely, effective goals are specific, divided into subgoals, and challenging (Locke & Latham, 2002). In contrast, ambiguous goals such as "do your best" function about the same as not setting goals at all. This is interesting because it is common for adults to tell learners to do their best. That turns out to be poor advice because doing one's best is so vague as to function as no goal at all.

Specific components of effective goal setting are displayed in Table 2.1 and discussed below. Examples in Table 2.1 are given for an English speaker who wants to learn Spanish.

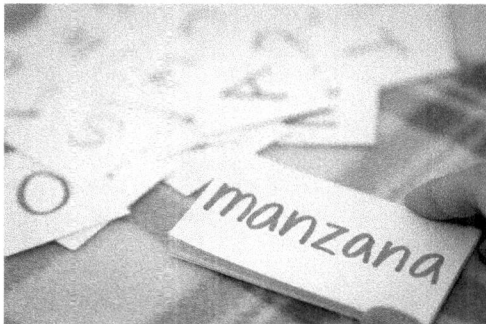

Specificity

It is relatively easy to think of specific goals for activities like getting a job (e.g., I will get this job) or running (e.g., I will achieve a 10-minute mile). However, generating specific goals for activities such as learning a new language, improving confidence, getting physically fit, or appreciating Shakespeare are more challenging because what constitutes mastery is less concrete. For some domains, specific goals can be framed in terms of time (e.g., I will study at least 30 minutes per day) and output (e.g., I will write at least 500 words per day).

Subgoals

Short-term sub-goals help learners make progress toward larger long-term goals. For example, a speech pathologist might work with a child who has

Table 2.1 Effective goal setting for an English speaker who wants to learn Spanish

Effective goal attributes	*Description*	*Example*
Specific	It is clear when the goal has been achieved.	*I want to be able to listen to Spanish tv without subtitles and converse with native Spanish speakers about my hobbies, current events, and movies.*
Long-term goal is divided into subgoals	Small steps scaffold the learner toward the long-term goal. The subgoals should follow a sequence and receive feedback.	*Each day I will view 15 minutes of Spanish language tv with subtitles and 15 minutes without subtitles. I will read a popular book in Spanish out loud for 10 minutes. I will converse 3 times a week for 20 minutes with my Mexican neighbor. I will use the Spanish app to learn the "word of the day."*
Challenging	Goals are appropriately challenging, that is, slightly beyond the person's current ability level, but not too difficult.	*The overall goal of learning Spanish is very difficult, but I can handle each of the subgoals.*
Involves feedback	A coach, teacher, expert, peer, or recording device (like video) provides feedback on goal progress and strategies for improvement.	*When I view tv without subtitles I will know if I am understanding. My neighbor will give me feedback about my accent and whether she can understand me.*
Highly committed	Learners are so committed to achieving the goal that they are willing to give up competing activities.	*I will give up some video game playing to free up time.*
Plan to overcome barriers	Learners devise strategies for self-regulation and plans to overcome stumbling blocks.	*I will probably be tempted to view subtitles, so I will tape a card over the tv screen where subtitles are displayed. It is embarrassing to speak bad Spanish with my neighbor, so I will bring snacks to make it more fun.*
Goals are shared	Share goals with someone of higher status, like a coach, teacher, or parent.	*I will write my goals and email them to my Spanish teacher.*

Note: Relevant works include the following: (Bergin & Prewett, 2020; Gollwitzer & Oettingen, 2012; Klein et al., 2020; Locke & Latham, 2002, 2006)

poor articulation. Subgoals might include reducing deletion of final consonants (saying *cu* instead of *cup*) and reducing palatal fronting (saying *soot* instead of *shoot*).

Challenge

Performance tends to rise when learners set goals that are challenging but realistically achievable with effort. For an introvert, making eight prospective job contacts per day might be quite challenging, but others might find it less challenging and set a higher subgoal.

Feedback

Feedback is information provided by a person or some other mechanism regarding one's performance. Feedback about progress toward goals helps learners know where they need to try harder. Feedback can come from others such as a coach, therapist, or instructor who describes where the learner is falling short. Feedback from charts and checklists helps learners check their progress. Teachers, therapists, and coaches can be tremendous assets for teaching how to keep charts and checklists. There are apps that track progress toward goals. Feedback can also be a natural consequence of going after a goal; solving a difficult math problem, getting a job interview, and improving articulation all provide feedback that you are on the path to success.

Goal Commitment

Achieving challenging goals takes effort. Learners are not likely to achieve goals unless they are committed to the toil required. Learners are more likely to commit to goals if they view the goals as important and attainable (Locke & Latham, 2002). They need to feel competent enough to attain the goal; if they feel that they lack relevant ability, they are likely to quit. Goal commitment is influenced by peers. If learners feel that their peers are committed to the same goal, they are more likely to commit themselves. Note that it can be easy to get learners to *say* that they are committed to a goal; it is much more difficult to achieve true commitment.

When a learner has multiple goals, one goal can pull resources away from another goal. For example, a teen might have a goal to get into a top university and a conflicting goal to work long hours and contribute financially to the family; each goal requires time that must be taken away from pursuit of the other goal. Teachers, parents, coaches, therapists and other authority figures should be aware of the possibility of conflicting goals and have strategies to address the issue. This issue comes up when children and youth are pursuing time consuming extra-curricular activities that conflict with schoolwork (and sleep). While participation in extra-curricular activities is positively correlated with achievement, in individual cases that might not be true. Learners should be counseled about how to balance goals.

Goal commitment can also be problematic when therapist goals and client goals do not match. For example, a study of people with aphasia, an impairment in using and understanding written or spoken language, found that clients and therapists did not always have the same goals (Rohde et al., 2012). Clients tended to focus more than therapists on returning to activities that they enjoyed. Clients are less committed to goals that therapists impose. Collaboration in goal setting is one way to foster goal commitment, but collaboration is particularly difficult with clients who suffer from language impairment.

Plan to Overcome Barriers

The most successful goal setters have strategies for overcoming barriers and difficulties (Gollwitzer & Sheeran, 2006). For example, learners are surrounded with temptations when studying. One study found that when college students attempted to study alone for three hours, they tended to divert their attention to checking their cell phones, reading emails, looking at websites unrelated to their studying, and so forth, hardly a recipe for effective study (Calderwood et al., 2014). Learners should anticipate obstacles (e.g., the urge to check messages while studying) and create a contingency "if-then" plan. For example, "If I feel lost in a section of my statistics course, I will read relevant sections in two additional textbooks, and I will attend tutoring sessions." Studies have investigated goals to eat more fruits and vegetables. Participants were asked to write action plans for situations that might prevent them from eating fruits and vegetables and how they would respond (Kreausukon et al., 2012; Luszczynska et al., 2007).

Research shows that if-then plans help people overcome obstacles and achieve their goals. If-then plans should attempt to create automaticity, that is, when a particular situation is encountered, specific responses are automatically activated. This reduces the difficulty of decision making in-the-moment—shall I do this or this? Instead, the decision has already been made, and the person merely needs to automatically follow the pre-made decision.

Be Strategic

Sometimes when people set goals, they come up with an approach to completing the goal and stick with it. But sometimes the approach is ineffective, which should be obvious if the goal setter stopped to think about it. But often they do not. A study of strategic mindset found that learners who spontaneously stop and ask themselves if they are going about goal pursuit in the most efficient and effective way possible reported higher grades and greater progress toward their personal goals in the areas of profession, education, health, and fitness. The researchers randomly assigned an intervention group that was taught to ask themselves "How else can I do this? Are there things that I can do differently? Are there ways to do this even better?" (Chen et al., 2020, p. 14069). The strategic questioning group practiced more, used more varied strategies, and ended up with higher performance than the control group. Another study using similar methods improved the grades of students (Chen et al., 2017). You can encourage your goal setters to ask themselves if they are using the best techniques or could they improve. You can tailor your prompts to the situation with questions such as "What are your available resources?" "Are you using those resources?" and "Who could you ask for feedback?"

Personal Best Goal

A different way of thinking about goal setting is to set a personal best goal (Martin & Elliot, 2016). Domains that have clear, measured outcomes lend themselves to this sort of goal setting because the goals are easily specified. For example, a student could set a goal of getting a personal best score on an exam or a personal best time on a race. However, personal best goals can also apply to the *process* of achieving a goal. For example, a student could set a goal of studying intensely for more hours than in the past, or making more kind comments to a sibling, or doing more revisions of a manuscript. An advantage of personal best goals is that the learner is focused on personal improvement rather than comparison with others; this invokes mastery goals and growth mindset, both of which tend to foster well-being. In one study elementary and secondary students set a personal best goal to score better than they had the previous year on a standardized test. Note that they set the goal while they still had time to study for the test; they scored better than a control group (see Figure 2.1, Martin & Elliot, 2016).

Incentives

Many people believe that incentives like money provide goals that students desire and will successfully pursue. In some situations, incentives can work, but generally they do not work well. In a massive series of field experiments with random assignment, researchers paid students in over 200 schools in Dallas, New York, and Chicago for grades, to read books, and for interim assessments (Fryer, 2011). They distributed $9.4 million to roughly 27,000 students. They found zero effect overall. They conjectured that the pattern of results across cities suggests that when students are paid

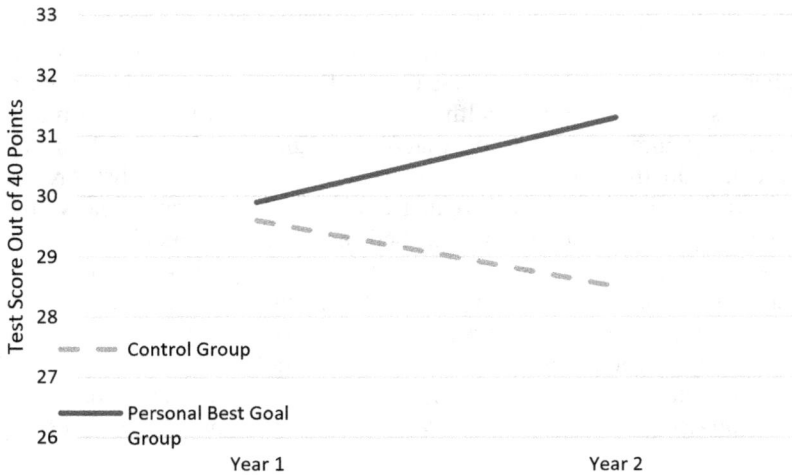

Figure 2.1 Adapted from Martin & Elliot, 2016.

for test scores, they don't have a clear idea of what strategies to use to achieve the desired test scores and get the money. In New York, researchers interviewed a subset of students and asked what they could do to earn more money on the next test (Fryer, 2010). Students struggled to answer. Those who answered focused on test-taking strategies like reading the items more carefully. Not a single student said that they should study more, read the book more carefully, ask teachers about confusing topics, or complete their homework. The study did find that students in Dallas who were not English Language Learners and who were paid to read books had significantly higher reading test scores. When the Dallas students were paid to read, they did not have to think about strategies because reading contributed directly to improved test scores and the students didn't have to figure out strategies. They were paid to do the thing that results in higher test scores.

Other studies confirm that paying or providing overt incentives for performance has little effect (Bergin et al., 2007; O'Neil et al., 2005; O'Neil et al., 1995/1996; Slavin, 2010; Spencer et al., 2005). In fact, in one study in India, where a little money goes farther than in the US, very high financial incentives had a detrimental effect on performance (Ariely et al., 2009). The message for those who work with youth is to not rely upon rewards, money, or other incentives to provide goals.

Additional Suggestions for Goal Setting

The following are additional suggestions for helping learners set goals:

- *Provide explicit instruction for setting goals.* Don't assume that you can just tell young people to set goals. They need to be taught how. Refer to Table 2.1 as you guide youth to set specific goals, making sure they are measurable. Figuring out how to set meaningful goals in some domains takes considerable thought; how will you know if your students appreciate Shakespeare, can recognize symbolism in literature, or have improved their self-confidence? Those goals are challenging to specify and measure. Part of teaching others to set goals is helping them break down long-term goals into smaller, short-term sub-goals. For example, if an athlete wants to improve for a specific sport, goals could involve weight training, aerobic training, and practice; each of those domains can have short-term and long-term goals.
- *Help learners set appropriately challenging goals.* While having learners set their own goals can be useful because it can enhance commitment to the goals, it is not the only way. Children and youth often respect therapists, coaches, or teachers and believe that these adults have insight into the goal setter's capabilities; goal setters often benefit when those respected guides help set the goals. You can use your expertise to persuade learners that challenging goals are important and attainable and to help set the appropriate level of challenge (Locke et al., 1988).
- *Regularly monitor progress.* Goal setters benefit from tracking their progress. Help them set up spreadsheets, apps, or checklists to track the short-term and long-term goals.
- *Encourage sharing goals publicly and with someone of higher status.* Sharing goals publicly can increase performance (Epton et al., 2017). Sharing goals with someone of higher status, like a coach, teacher, therapist, administrator, or parent, can increase goal commitment and goal achievement (Klein et al., 2020).

Research and Theory into Practice

A study of struggling college students investigated goal setting (Morisano et al., 2010). The 85 students had GPAs below 3.0. Students were randomly assigned to the intervention or to a control group. The intervention was a single online activity that took about 2.5 uninterrupted hours. The students were asked to write about their ideal future, list areas for improvement, generate specific goals, rank the goals, write strategies for achieving goals, and describe how they would know if a goal was achieved. The goal setting session improved grades significantly, from 2.25 to 2.91, over an academic year (see Figure 2.2). This is something that parents, teachers, or therapists could try with youth to help them think about their futures and their goals.

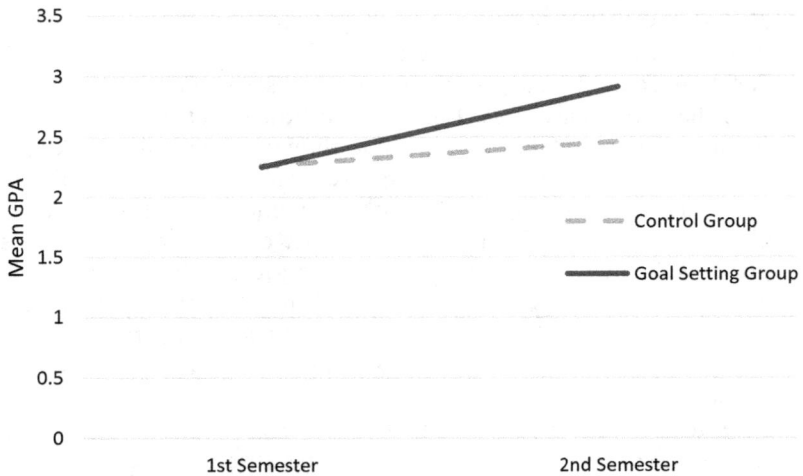

Figure 2.2 Adapted from Morisano et al., 2010.

Another approach to the same sort of goal setting and goal clarification comes from Ford and Nichols' (1991) assessment of core goals. You set aside several hours and start by writing a list of past experiences that were exceptionally satisfying or enjoyable. Then you examine the list and try to identify for each experience the moment of peak satisfaction and the specific event that triggered that feeling. This leads to a search for common underlying themes. Group together experiences that seem to have produced the same or a similar outcome. Your aim is to generate a list of your own core goals, things like fostering family closeness, providing help to others, experiencing the out-of-doors, winning competitions, generating creative art works, and so forth. Once you have that list, you can be more mindful in choosing experiences and modifying experiences so that they fit your core goals. Let's say that you have children and find that family closeness is a core goal. When you next have an out-of-town conference, you could take one child with you and have some special outings with that child. On the other hand, if getting ahead in your career is a core goal, taking a child on a business trip might be a distraction.

Interview: Rewards and Incentives

Early Childhood Teacher at a Rural School. Three Years of Experience

One concept that really stood out to me was rewards and motivation in students, specifically young students. One concept that specifically stuck out to me was that the use of tangible rewards may undermine students' intrinsic motivation. I began to think about the reading log system that we use at the early learning center where I teach. Each month, every student in the school gets a "reading log" that they color in each time they read for 20 minutes at home. Once their log is all the way colored in, they bring it to school and get to pick out a prize with our school principal. At the beginning of the year, I notice that my students are SO excited to work on their reading logs and bring them to school for a prize. They'll talk about it constantly with their peers and will run in my classroom door shouting, "Ms. ___, look what I finished!" However, by the end of the school year, this is not the case. Students don't feel nearly as excited to pick out prizes (because the prize bucket rarely gets new toys in it); therefore, they don't really care to bring in their reading logs anymore. The same concept relates to one of my teacher friends who also teaches at my school. She has a system set up in her room where when students are kind, they get stickers and eventually get to go to the treasure chest when their sticker charts are all the way filled up. However, she often tells me that she notices students are only being kind to one another when the teacher is looking (situational compliance). After a while, they also get tired of the toys and no longer care about their sticker sheets.

Kids do Well If They Can

Sometimes adults think that certain children don't care about learning or doing well, particularly in school. It is important to verify that the children have the competence to do what is asked. Sometimes children want to follow instructions but lack the ability. Ross Greene (2008) pointed out that kids *do well if they can*, but many adults believe that *kids only do well if they want to*. Thus, many adults believe that if kids are doing poorly, it is because they lack motivation and don't want to do well rather than because they lack necessary skills. Therefore, adults reward and punish rather than teaching. They may say that the children just want attention, want their own way, are manipulating, are not motivated, have incompetent parents, or have a bad attitude. Greene listed things that children might have trouble with such as understanding instruction, handling transitions, generating the motivation to persist on boring tasks, keeping track of time, maintaining focus, anticipating consequences of behavior, and being nice. Rather than punishing them for something they cannot do, it would be better to figure out what is the problem.

Greene (2010) advocates a three-step process:

1   *Empathy* step. Gather information about the problem from the child's perspective. Say something like, "I have noticed that you _____" where you fill in the blank with the behavior, such as "I have noticed

that you don't seem to be understanding algebra" or "I have noticed that you consistently tease your classmate." Then ask, "What's up?" Adults often assume that they already know "What's up," so they might not listen well. They need to drop their assumptions and listen.

2   *Define the problem* step. State how the problem is affecting the child and/or other people. "When you don't understand the algebra now, you will have increasing difficulty with future material." "When you come in late, you disrupt other students and you miss instruction."

3   *Invitation* step. The adult and child jointly discuss possible solutions that address the problems.

Greene (2010) gives the example of a male principal who has the problem of a student who is fighting on the bus. If he merely forbids fighting and imposes penalties, he is not likely to solve the problem. He discovers that the student is being taunted by another student. The principal may be tempted to suggest ignoring the taunting, a typical but doomed adult suggestion. He may recommend putting the student on another bus, a solution that ignores the underlying problem and has logistical problems like how do you find another bus that goes to the correct place. If he follows Greene's process, he will invite

> the student to solve the problem collaboratively. Instead of *deciding* what's going to happen—'I'm going to put you on a different bus'—he *wonders* what will happen: 'I'm wondering whether there's a way for you two to work out your bad blood?' Then he and the student come up with a plan to begin solving the problem together.
>
> (p. 33)

Greene calls his approach Collaborative & Proactive Solutions (CPS, formerly called Collaborative Problem Solving).

Collaborative & Proactive Solutions improves the relationship between staff, students, and parents. It also helps students trust adults and helps teachers feel that they can assist their students.

Experiences with Goals

When one considers goals, it is important to consider their complexity. For example, a youth might be on a sports team because of goals to spend time with friends or to please parents rather than for love of the sport. Other possible goals include impressing friends, becoming physically fit, getting to travel with the team, and so forth. It is important to consider the multiplicity of possible goals so that you don't jump to assumptions about students' goals. For example, I once observed MathCounts practices and competitions. MathCounts is a nationwide math competition for students Grades 6–8 that takes place outside of school time. People I talked with seemed to assume that students in MathCounts were intrinsically motivated to learn about math. Not necessarily so. When I talked with students and their parents, I found that some students did like math, but some participated primarily to be with friends, to please parents, or because their parents required them to participate. MathCounts coaches needed to consider varied motivations, not just liking math. If being with friends is an important goal for MathCounts participants, having students sit in rows and do solitary math worksheets will leave learners feeling dissatisfied. Leaders in all domains should consider the learners' varied goals and address them as appropriate.

It is important to question assumptions when addressing goals. For example, teachers often have a goal that parents read to their children at home. One teacher wrote about his experience with a poor reader, Ronny (Done, 2005). Ronny did not read with his parents, so the teacher sent a note to his mother explaining the importance of reading with children. He also sent some picture books like *Curious George* and *Frog and Toad*. He would ask Ronny if his mother had read to him the night before, and Ronny always said that she was too busy. The teacher assumed the mother was not interested in improving her son's learning. Then one day the teacher noticed that Ronny's mother was at the school for an adult education class. He complained to another teacher that Ronny's mom wouldn't help her son improve his reading but would take a pottery class. The other teacher stared at him and said that Ronny's mother was there to take a beginning reading class because she did not know how to read. The teacher realized that Ronny's mother did not have a lack-of-motivation-to-read-to-her-son problem, she had a don't-know-how-to-read problem. His assumptions were wrong, he had been judging her unfairly, and his intervention had been inappropriate. Later, Ronny's mother thanked the teacher and said, "I'm grateful that you sent all those books home every night with Ronny. Thank you, Mr. Done. You helped me learn to read" (p. 67). Like Ross Greene's students who want to do well but lack skills, this parent had a goal to help her son but lacked the skills.

Educators need to be aware of dimensions of the environment that affect students' ability to pursue educational goals. It might be simple to recommend that students use the public library as a resource. But what if the students don't have transportation? Worse, what if the library is in another gang's turf? A principal in New York City wrote,

> Kids from Seth Low or Howard Houses can't come to this community center. It's a death sentence if they do. And the library? If you tell the kids they have to go to the library, some of them can't even cross over

to go there, because then they would be traveling into another gang's area. We often don't think about those things.

(Lopez, 2016, p. 179)

The podcast *This American Life* included a two-part show about Harper High School on the south side of Chicago (*This American Life*, 2013). The neighborhood was so violent that the previous year, 29 students had been shot. It was difficult for students to pursue educational goals when they were just trying to survive. When administrators talked with kids, one of the first things they tried to figure out was where the kids lived and which gang controlled that territory. It was dangerous to walk alone because youth could be attacked, but it was also dangerous to walk with a group because they could be labeled as part of a gang and attacked. Educators need to be aware of this sort of neighborhood dynamic so that they can make reasonable requests of students about collaborating with fellow students and attending events. Students may avoid certain activities not for lack of motivation, but for safety.

Teachers, therapists, coaches, and parents, should carefully consider children's goals as they attempt to foster children's well-being. What goals does a child have? Where do the goals come from? Are they adaptive? What can adults do to support goal achievement?

Summary

- A goal is an intention to achieve future valued outcomes.
- Goals are influenced by families, SES, culture, peers, teachers, therapists, and coaches.
- Achievement goals include

    a   Mastery approach goals: striving to improve skills and understand. They are linked with deeper learning strategies, low anxiety, preference for challenging tasks, intrinsic motivation, and relatively high performance.
    b   Performance approach goals: striving to demonstrate ability and to do better than others. They are linked with high performance, relatively high anxiety, and concern with appearance.
    c   Performance avoidance goals: striving to avoid appearing unable and doing worse than others. They are linked with low achievement, high anxiety, and concern with appearance.

- Growth mindset refers to a belief that ability can be developed through effort and effective strategies. A growth mindset is more adaptive than a fixed mindset, which refers to a belief that ability is fixed and unchangeable.
- Goal setting consistently improves performance in most domains.

- Effective goals have the following attributes

  a Specific
  b Divided into subgoals
  c Challenging
  d Involve feedback
  e High level of commitment
  f Include a plan to overcome barriers
  g Goals are shared

- Incentives like paying for grades generally do not work well for motivating learning.
- Kids do well if they can, but sometimes they lack the skills to do well. Effective intervention then involves teaching skills.

Suggestions for Further Reading

Dweck, C. S. (2006). *Mindset: The New Psychology of Success.* Random House.

Greene, R. (2008). Kids do well if they can. *Phi Delta Kappan, 90*(3), 160–167.

Greene, R. (2011). Collaborative problem solving can transform school discipline. *Phi Delta Kappan, 93*(2), 25–29.

Locke, E. A., & Latham, G. P. (1984). *Goal Setting: A Motivational Technique that Works!* Prentice-Hall.

Locke, E. A., & Latham, G. P. (2002). Building a practically useful theory of goal setting and task motivation: A 35-year odyssey. *American Psychologist, 57*(9), 705–717.

Chapter 3

Do Children and Youth Feel Competent?

Understanding and Influencing Self-Efficacy and Motivation

John Thompson, the championship-winning basketball player and coach, wrote that when he was a child, he was labeled stupid and "retarded" (Thompson, 2020, p. 20). He felt he was labeled because he was Black. When he was in sixth grade, his teacher told him, "You're not stupid. You just can't read." His teacher and mother took him to various reading specialists until they found one who helped. The specialist happened to be Black. Thompson learned to read. He wrote, "most of the white people I had encountered in the educational system up to that point in my life thought I was 'retarded.' You can read that however you want to" (p. 22). Once he had the skills to read, he became competent in the classroom, which fostered his academic efficacy and motivation to succeed academically, though he admits that he was more interested in basketball than in achieving high grades.

Feeling competent is a key component of motivation. For example, students who achieve low grades in math are less likely to continue studying mathematics than students with high grades (Brown et al., 2008); this finding seems so obvious as to hardly merit mentioning. When asked if they intended to continue studying mathematics, some 16-year-olds wrote statements like

> "Its just too damn hard."
> "Everyone who I have spoken to who is on the course says it is way too hard and is not worth it."
> "I hate mathematics and I would rather die."
>
> (pp. 7, 10)

Even some high achievers had doubts about their competence such as the student who said, "I don't feel confident enough to do so even if I'm at an A grade" (p. 12).

Concerns about competence are big for high school students. One study (Wentzel et al., 2019) asked students to write what most concerned them as they transitioned from eighth grade to high school, again in ninth grade, and again in tenth grade. In all three grades, the most common

DOI: 10.4324/9781003046516-3

concerns were about competence. Examples included ability to maintain good grades, score well on tests, manage the workload, qualify for extra-curricular activities, stay safe and stay out of trouble. Understanding the development of perceptions of competence and actual competence are key for educators, therapists, and coaches.

Sometimes adults who have mastered a skill like reading, interacting socially, or driving a car forget how difficult it is to learn a new skill. In fact, some adults avoid learning new skills because it is so difficult and potentially embarrassing. A teacher educator required her aspiring teachers to learn—or at least attempt to learn—how to juggle (Knowles, 2021). She meant real juggling of beanbags, not metaphorical juggling of tasks. After attempting to learn to juggle, one student reported,

> I understand what it is like to be the child learning the new task, being frustrated with the task, ready to give up, and wanting to do away with the objects causing the frustration. I realized what it was like to make excuses for myself as to why I could not learn this new skill.

Another student said,

> This activity has opened my eyes to the world of teaching. I stood in my future students' shoes and saw what they deal with every day. Now that I have the reminder of how difficult it can be to learn something new, I will be a better teacher.
>
> (p. 58).

Acquiring competence can be motivating for student *and* teacher. Barbara LoMonaco was teaching math to second graders. In subtraction, Annabelle could not grasp tens and ones with borrowing or regrouping. She looked blank and confused. Ms. LoMonaco tried using charts to illustrate place value, then ice cream sticks rubber-banded into groups of tens and ones, then beans, sparkly stones, and pretzels. Nothing worked. Then, one day while tutoring Annabelle after school, she used the same approaches again. Annabelle got quiet, stopped squirming, took a deep breath, and smiled. They cheered and hugged and ate pretzels. Ms. LoMonaco felt competent as a teacher, able to teach, and Annabelle felt competent as a learner, able to subtract with regrouping. Both increased in motivation.

Self-Efficacy

A competence concept that has been extensively studied is self-efficacy (Bandura, 1997), which refers to individuals' beliefs in their ability to exert control over themselves and their environment. Self-efficacy refers to their perceptions of their own competence to *do things* (e.g., can I write an effective paper about *Romeo and Juliet?*) and to *control their own thinking* (e.g., can I control my thoughts even when I am bored or distracted?). Self-efficacy is usually framed as specific to a domain, topic, or skill like math, art, or sports (Bandura, 2012). Domains can be fairly broad, such as math efficacy or ability to regulate anxious thoughts, or they can be more limited, such as efficacy for algebra or efficacy for shooting free throws. Students often have high efficacy for some academic domains, like literature and music, but low efficacy for other domains, like math and physics.

Self-efficacy influences motivation to learn and pursue activities because people avoid domains for which they feel incompetent. Students who are unathletic and get teased when the class goes outside to play sports are likely to develop low self-efficacy for sports. They may develop strategies to avoid situations that highlight their weak sports ability like volunteering to help out in the school office or suddenly having a headache.

The importance of self-efficacy is not limited to youth. Teachers who have high efficacy tend to use more effective teaching strategies, demonstrate better classroom management, and experience less burnout compared with low efficacy teachers (Zee & Koomen, 2016). Teachers with high efficacy believe that they can reach even difficult students, accurately assess how much their students are learning, increase learning of students whose families are unsupportive, and adjust instruction to engage failing students. Counselors with high efficacy believe they can reach even difficult clients, show empathy towards clients, and help clients figure out what triggers their substance use.

Self-efficacy is foundational to success in many domains. Interventions with chronic disease patients show that self-efficacy is a key element of disease self-management (Marks & Allegrante, 2005). Young people with chronic disease need efficacy that they can monitor correct medication, engage in exercise, select appropriate foods, and use stress management strategies even in the face of challenging situations like holiday activities. Type 1 and Type 2 diabetes are examples of diseases that afflict youth and are difficult to manage (Hilliard et al., 2016). Youth with Type 2 diabetes typically also experience obesity, which means both the disease and weight should be managed. Interventions often include self-efficacy for self-management in their protocols.

Learners with high self-efficacy are confident that they can be successful. When they encounter barriers or failure, they are likely to develop strategies for overcoming them. They blame failure on internal factors such as poor preparation or external factors such as bad teaching or bad luck rather than their own lack of innate ability. They feel confident that given another try and more practice, they can succeed. Learners with high academic efficacy who do poorly on an exam don't give up. They study harder for the next exam and seek help. They look for the next opportunity to show what they can do. In contrast, learners with low self-efficacy avoid challenging tasks and quit after a failure because they view additional effort as fruitless.

Recall that effective goal setting requires goal commitment. Self-efficacy is necessary for goal commitment. Learners with high efficacy are not afraid to commit to difficult goals. Because learners with greater self-efficacy are more likely to persevere through challenges, they are then more likely to achieve their goals.

Children and youth with low efficacy may be motivated to engage in self-handicapping, which refers to behaviors that allow you to excuse failure and that give you extra credit for success. These behaviors can protect the ego but undermine learning and achievement. One behavior is avoiding high effort. If you try hard and fail, it suggests you are not competent, which makes you feel bad. If you don't try and fail, it is less threatening to the ego. In school settings, self-handicappers might skip doing homework so that when they get low grades, they can defend their ego by saying that they didn't even try. Additional self-handicapping strategies in school settings include procrastinating, fooling around instead of studying, claiming illness or anxiety, and pursuing lots of activities so that there is little time for studying. Not surprisingly, self-handicapping predicts lower achievement (Schwinger et al., 2014). In sports settings, self-handicapping includes avoiding practice and feigning illness. The book *The Sports Gene* (Epstein, 2013) gives the example of an 800-meter runner who had not been running well; he told his teammate that he was going to drop out of a race at 600 meters, apparently in order to protect his ego. If he did not even finish the race, he would not have to explain to himself (and others) why he lost.

It is also interesting that children and youth may *claim* that they did not try hard when in fact they did. Athletes with low efficacy may not want to sabotage their own performance by not practicing, but they can protect their ego by claiming to have had weak practices or sore joints. We all know people who have claimed to have forgotten an assignment until the last minute, to have slacked off in sports practice, or to have been ill—all in order to reduce expectations of high performance. But if by chance they achieved high performance, they glowed in the implication that they had very high ability because they did not prepare well but still performed well.

Research describes four influences on the development of self-efficacy (Bandura, 1997). *Mastery experience*, or previous success, is usually the most powerful. Just learning skills is not enough; learners need to enact their skills. After a learning experience, people think about whether they can replicate successes and improve upon failures. The more successes they have and skills they learn, the greater the self-efficacy they develop. An interview study of middle school math students found that students with high efficacy reported high grades, high test scores, and high effort.

Strong academic performance seemed to go hand-in-hand with confidence. Zach and Hannah were quick to point out that they had never earned below a high A average in math. Each beamed about having outperformed others on standardized tests.

(Usher, 2009, p. 289)

In contrast, students with low self-efficacy reported declining grades and disappointing performance. For example, Xavier had never received an F on his report card until he was in seventh grade math, and when he got the F, "I just shut down. I just quit believing in myself" (p. 292). Xavier's beliefs in his mathematical competence were shattered. He adopted a fixed mindset that he was not competent in math: "It's just so hard. I, I don't think I'm smart enough for it or something" (p. 292).

A second influence on self-efficacy is *vicarious experience*. Individuals watch others who are successful or unsuccessful and use that information to assess their own probability of success. This vicarious experience allows them to assess their own level of competence. A student wrote that they did not want to study more math because "My sister found A2 maths very hard and her frustration with it persuaded me not to study it" (Brown et al., 2008, p. 7). Jennifer Doudna, who won the 2020 Nobel Prize in chemistry, said that when she read the book *The Double Helix* as a 6th grader, the scientist Rosalind Franklin jumped out for her because she was a woman and was a great scientist—"reading the book was the first time I really thought about it, and it was an eye-opener. Women could be scientists" (Isaacson, 2021, p. 8). This vicarious experience bolstered her efficacy for science and put Doudna on track to become a great scientist herself.

Peer models are particularly effective at influencing self-efficacy. Learners say to themselves, "if that person who is similar to me can do it, I can do it, and if they cannot, I probably cannot either." An elementary teacher said, regarding teaching mathematics, "The professor shared her mathematics anxiety experiences with us and I felt like I could relate to her immediately. If she can overcome, I can overcome" (Gresham, 2018, p. 100).

Coping models are also effective for vicariously enhancing efficacy; coping models show how to cope with and overcome difficulty. A client who struggles with substance abuse might see others who faced similar struggles and who gradually overcame; viewing these coping models is likely to increase self-efficacy to avoid substance abuse: "If they can overcome, so can I, and I can imitate the strategies they used."

A third influence is *persuasion,* which occurs when other people persuade learners that they are (or are not) capable. Persuasion is usually most powerful coming from an expert. Compare your mother telling you that you are a great singer with a professional recording producer telling you. Who would influence your efficacy more? It is much more energizing when a tough teacher says that you are good than when friends or parents, who are expected to be nice, say that you are good. When a critical teacher says that you have the skills to pursue some activity or career, you really take notice. The same can happen in reverse. It is an unforgettable event when someone in authority says that you lack the skills to pursue some activity. A student wrote that they did not want to take more math because "I have been told by teachers it is too difficult for me" (Brown et al., 2008, p 7). Statements like, "You will never overcome substance use" or "Not everyone can be good at math" should never be uttered.

An adult wrote about his experience with persuasion back when he was in high school (Groendes, 2017). He wrote that he was faced with taking the easy English class or the difficult English class. He figured he was college-bound, so he chose the difficult class with Mrs. McDougal. One day, Mrs. McDougal called him out of class and told him that he was a promising writer and that he should submit his work for publication. He did go on to write successfully. At his 50th reunion, he discovered that Mrs. McDougal had taken various students aside and encouraged them to follow some talent that she had observed.

Michael Lewis, the famous author of *The Big Short*, was a bench warmer in a key high school baseball game and never expected to play in the game (Lewis, 2004). His team was up 2 to 1, but in the last inning, Lewis had to pitch in place of the star pitcher, and the other team danced with joy. They knew they could get hits off of Lewis. Coach Fitz handed Lewis the ball.

> I looked at their players, hugging and mugging and dancing and jeering. No, they did not appear to suspect that I was going to put [the ball] anywhere unpleasant. Then Fitz leaned down, put his hand on my shoulder and, thrusting his face right up to mine, became as calm as the eye of a storm. It was just him and me now; we were in this together. I have no idea where the man's intention ended and his instincts took over, but the effect of his performance was to say, There's no one I'd rather have out here in this life-or-death situation. And I believed him!

Lewis picked off the runner at third base and struck out the batter. The game was over, and he had won. Persuasion from a respected expert. It works.

The fourth influence on self-efficacy is *physiological states* such as anxiety and fatigue. Our emotions and the sweat on our palms tell us how confident we should be about sinking the free throw that would win the game. Consider someone who wants to go cliff jumping, but when they look down from the cliff, their suddenly rapid heartbeat tells them that they might smack the water very hard in the wrong places. Their confidence plumets. The same thing can happen when students walk to the front of the class to solve a difficult problem or see a test item that they don't understand.

Efficacy Interventions

Changing self-efficacy changes behavior. For example, a meta-analysis found that improving people's self-efficacy that they can change their health-related behavior indeed promotes positive change (Sheeran et al., 2016). The study analyzed experimental interventions with random assignment to control groups. Behaviors that were studied included adolescent safe sex intentions, junior high sexual intercourse postponement, smoking cessation, elementary school seatbelt and bike helmet use, childhood obesity, sugar reduction in children, physical activity, eating vegetables, and others. These results make clear that it is important for teachers, coaches, and therapists to think about what might be influencing their learners' and clients' self-efficacy and how they can raise self-efficacy.

You can influence learners' self-efficacy in at least four ways that parallel the sources of self-efficacy. First, you should foster mastery experience by providing high-quality instruction so that most learners and clients learn skills and then experience success. For learners who struggle, this may require taking them aside for one-on-one tutoring. Care should be taken not to embarrass learners by paying excessive attention to them publicly; such attention can mark them as less competent and undermine attempts to improve their efficacy. Providing unsolicited help can also backfire by communicating to the learner that he or she needs extra help that others do not need.

Second, instructors can provide vicarious experience through models, especially peer models or near peer models. For example, a high school teacher could invite recent graduates to visit the school and describe their experiences finding jobs, working in the military, or going to college. A substance abuse therapist could invite former addicts who have been clean and are willing to talk about their experiences. Models can be live or virtual. They can be in books, magazines, or videos. High school athletes often watch professionals and listen to their after-game comments; they enhance their efficacy by learning "what the pro's do." People making home repairs may feel intimidated by the task until they watch a couple of YouTube videos that show what to do and how; such vicarious models can substantially enhance efficacy.

Third, instructors can use persuasion and tell learners that they are capable, or have credible significant others do so. For example, cross-country coach Diljeet Taylor, whose team won the 2020 NCAA title, said that her high school coach gave her an encouraging note before a meet. She found the notes so useful that she gives hand-written notes to her own athletes before each meet (Kuzma, 2019). This sort of encouraging word can help youth see themselves as efficacious and confident. Adults can also point out times in the past when learners were successful. "Remember the time you got an A on your math test?" or "Remember when you used your breathing strategies and made your anxiety go away?"

Finally, instructors can structure learning environments to avoid negative physiological states like anxiety. For example, they can avoid time limits that tend to make learners feel stressed. They can also help learners re-interpret anxiety as "excitement" rather than "fear" (Brooks, 2014). For example, learners can use self-talk such as saying "I am excited" out loud. A teacher can tell them to get excited. This is a different approach from suggesting that anxious students should try to calm themselves with breathing or other techniques. Both anxiety and excitement mean that a person will experience increased heart rate. It is more difficult to reduce the heart rate, as calming would require, compared to simply acknowledging that the heart is beating fast and labeling it as excitement. In addition, excitement is an approach emotion, meaning that it suggests that you should engage the task while anxiety is an avoidance emotion, meaning that you should avoid the task.

Mere education is not an effective intervention—merely knowing skills is not likely to change behavior. Children and youth need to try out skills and feel resilient efficacy that they have the skills to cope with the challenges that they face. Interventionists often combine influences on self-efficacy. For example, an intervention to increase eating fruits and vegetables asked participants to recall a time when they decided not to eat less healthy food and to eat or drink something more healthy (Luszczynska et al., 2007). They were asked to feel proud that they had stuck to their decision to eat more healthy food. This intervention invoked mastery experience, persuasion, and self-as-model.

Mastery modeling involves participants viewing a successful model and then enacting the behavior until they have success. This combines mastery experience, modeling, persuasion from the instructor, and learning to control physiological responses. An intervention to increase condom use (Bryan et al., 1996) had young adult women role play what to say to their partner; this combined simulated mastery experience, modeling through observing what others said, persuasion from the instructor, and learning to control feelings of anxiety and embarrassment.

Case 3.1

I was hiking in a rustic park with a group of 8 13-year-old boys. We came upon a wooden frame about 12 feet high with a thick rope hanging down. It was apparently an exercise apparatus for rope climbing. The boys started swinging on the rope. I said, "That rope is not for swinging. It is for climbing," and I climbed the rope and tapped the top crossbar. (See Figure 3.1.) Of course, each boy then wanted to climb the rope. A 13-year-old climbed half-way up and gave up. Then his ten-year-old brother slowly climbed to the top and tapped the crossbar. What do you think the 13-year-old did? Why? How are self-efficacy and influences on self-efficacy relevant? [You guessed it! The 13-year-old immediately climbed to the top. Had his skills changed in five minutes? No. He saw that his brother could do it and said to himself, "If my little brother can do it, I can do it." His self-efficacy changed in an instant through peer coping modeling.]

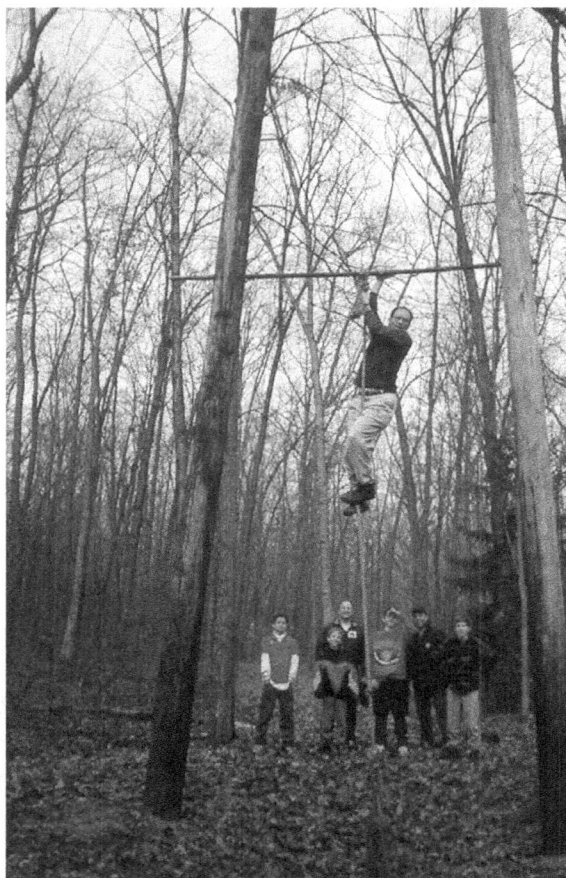

Figure 3.1

Overcoming Anxiety and Negative Emotions

Anxiety is pernicious and messes up working memory (Beilock, 2008). Working memory is where conscious thinking occurs, and it has limited capacity. When someone is solving problems, they are pulling information from their long-term memory and mixing that with incoming information from the environment. They might see a math problem (incoming information from the environment) and then try to pull relevant algorithms from their memory that would help them solve the problem. If they are anxious, their anxious thoughts mix in with the problem-solving information and make it difficult to solve the problems. "Let's see, if Max rides a bicycle up a hill at 20 miles per hour—*I am terrible at math and can never solve these kinds of problems*—and down the hill at 60 miles per hour—*who comes up with these stupid questions? This would never happen in the real world*—the distance is the same up and down. What is Max's average speed? This is an averaging problem so you take the two numbers, add them and divide by two—but that is too easy. This is supposed to be a difficult problem. *I don't know how to do math. I am terrible at math.* I guess I could just say 60+20=80 divided by 2 equals 40 so an average of 40 mph. *That is probably wrong but I don't care. Miles per hour is a ratio, so can you just add ratios and divide? This is too complicated for me.*" [40 is wrong. 30 is correct.] The anxious thoughts interfere with thinking about the problem. Students may have anxiety related to having observed or experienced violence, thinking about their parents' relationship problems, anticipating an exam, ruminating with peers about their own relationship problems, and so forth.

When students experience concerns about their competence, it can be useful to suggest that when they experience difficulty, it means that they are learning, not that they are failing (Autin & Croizet, 2012). Learning should be difficult, but students often interpret difficulty as an indication that they are *not* learning and that they lack the ability to do the task.

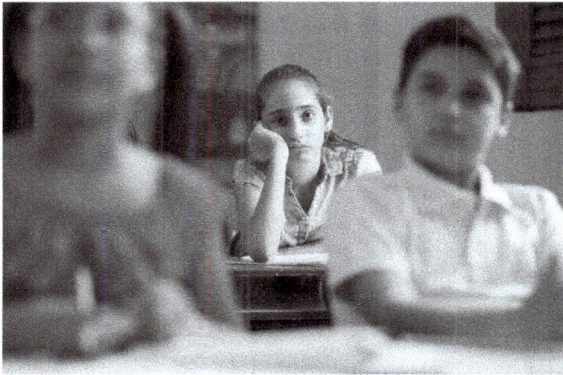

This can lead them to avoid learning tasks, which is self-defeating. So, a teacher, counselor, or psychologist can help them re-interpret their arousal and anxiety as an indication that they are learning.

Research and Theory into Practice

Teachers can suggest that anxiety helps performance. Researchers gave college students a 2.5 hour GRE practice test. A control group got generic instructions. The intervention group was told:

> People think that feeling anxious while taking a standardized test will make them do poorly on the test. However, recent research suggests that arousal doesn't hurt performance on these tests and can even help performance ... people who feel anxious during a test might actually do better. This means that you shouldn't feel concerned if you do feel anxious while taking today's GRE test. If you find yourself feeling anxious, simply remind yourself that your arousal could be helping you do well.
>
> (Jamieson et al., 2010, p. 209)

Results showed that the intervention group did better on the math section, though not on the verbal section (e.g., evaluation and comprehension of written material), of the practice GRE. Months later, the result was replicated: the intervention group did better on the math section, but not the verbal section, of the real GRE. The difference between math and verbal results could be that many students become more anxious about assessment of mathematical abilities compared to assessment of verbal abilities.

Brilliance and Perceptions of Competence

There is evidence that when students are led to believe that a field requires brilliance, females and African Americans are less likely to pursue that field. A study of 1820 faculty and graduate students at diverse research universities found that disciplines in which people believe that brilliance and innate giftedness are required for success had fewer women and African Americans (Leslie et al., 2015). Additional research supports this finding (Bian et al., 2018; Storage et al., 2020). This suggests that the way that adults talk about a field can influence the motivation of youth for that field. If adults suggest that a field requires a special aptitude that supposedly cannot be taught, they may turn away girls and students of color.

One way to combat the belief that a field is only for certain people is to teach how even apparently brilliant people struggled in their fields. If you have read educational stories about scientific discoveries or breakthroughs, you might have noticed that they tend to emphasize the brilliance of the scientists, who tend to be white and male. Stories about struggle rather than mere brilliance allow learners to connect with the narrative and think about the scientist as a model of effort as described by Bandura's self-efficacy research (coping models) and Dweck's mindset research (view ability as changeable through effort). One research study (Lin-Siegler et al., 2016) randomly assigned 9th and 10th grade students, predominantly low income and of color, to read stories about eminent scientists (Albert Einstein, Marie Curie, and Michael Faraday). There were three types of stories:

1   Scientist struggled and overcame mistakes, like coping models described earlier. The story was titled "Trying Over and Over Again Even When You Fail."
2   Scientist struggled in personal life such as overcoming poverty, fleeing the Nazis, or lacking family support. The story was titled "Overcoming the Challenges in Your Life."
3   Scientist was successful and no struggles were described (control condition). The story was titled "The Story of a Successful Scientist."

Results showed that students who read the struggle descriptions (numbers 1 and 2) improved their science learning compared to the control group. They reported feeling more connected to the struggling scientists compared to the no-struggle scientists. The description of Curie stated that because she was a woman, she had to study in secret and traveled from Poland to France because she was not permitted to study in Poland. One student wrote,

> I felt connected to Curie. Yes, I also went through an ordeal, when I first moved to U.S. There was only me and my mom in the country. We lived in a no heat apartment for one winter, everything in the room was frozen.
>
> (p. 322)

A follow-up to the scientist-struggle-study combined growth mindset, famous scientist struggle stories, and belonging mindset (Binning et al., 2019). Belonging mindset refers to helping students see that feeling left out can be normal and generally will go away as they meet and interact with new people. The study was done with 7th and 9th graders. The researchers chose to highlight academic and social struggles of famous celebrities (Oprah Winfrey, J.K. Rowling, Walt Disney, Daymond John) and scientists (Grace Murray Hopper, Neil deGrasse Tyson, Thomas Edison). In focus groups, the researchers verified that these celebrities and scientists were well-known by many students and had compelling adversity stories that would interest students. In addition, these celebrities and scientists represented different racial, gender, and SES groups. Interviews with students helped generate topics for belonging mindset testimonials in which students told about their own struggles in the schools that were being studied. A sample testimonial helped newcomers see that feeling out of place is normal and will change:

> When I got to 9th grade, everything felt different. All of my friends were changing and trying to be popular. Honestly, I thought I had to be just like them.... I had a hard time finding my real friends. But I realized a lot of people do too. I wish I could tell my 9th grade self, "Don't worry about fitting in! It takes time. Soon you'll find your group of friends."
>
> (p. 284)

Teachers, parents, and coaches can similarly tell about famous people and school peers who overcame adversity and excelled. This can be especially effective if the famous people and peers are from the same community and faced the same struggles as the children you are trying to influence.

Math Anxiety

Math anxiety undermines motivation and can be particularly difficult for students to deal with. Math anxiety can be communicated from parents. Research shows that parents with high math anxiety tend to have children with low math achievement, and their children learn less math than their peers. In one study, parents who had high math anxiety and tried to help frequently with math homework were particularly likely to reduce their children's learning (Maloney et al., 2015).

One intervention targeted parents who were math anxious (Schaeffer et al., 2018). The researchers had parents use an app with their children. The app started by presenting background information for a problem; for example, whipped cream was invented about 500 years ago by guys with unpronounceable Italian and French names. Then the app presented problems such as if one cup of heavy cream generates three cups of whipped cream, and if you whipped two cups of heavy cream, how many cups of air would you whip into the cream? Starting in 1st grade, the parents solved the problems with their children. The children's math achievement improved for the two years of the study.

Many studies have investigated expressive writing in which people write about events in their lives, especially traumatic or emotional events (Pennebaker & Chung, 2012). Such writing tends to have positive effects on well-being. A series of studies tested expressive writing used to reduce test anxiety before a major exam (Ramirez & Beilock, 2011). Ninth graders were asked to write essays before their first major biology exam in high school. Immediately before the exam, students were asked to write for ten minutes about their thoughts about the exam. Then they took the exam. There was also a control group. For the control group, the higher their test anxiety, the lower their score; that was not true for the expressive writing group, who outperformed the control group. The intervention was mainly effective for high test-anxious students. While the study was done with a biology exam, it seems likely to work equally well for other subjects like math.

Interview: Math Anxiety

5th and 6th grade Mathematics Teacher at a PreK–8th Grade Rural School. Eight Years of Experience

I know that some students have a dislike of math due to negative feedback and struggles, but I didn't realize that math anxiety was a real disorder until I encountered a sweet girl last year in my 5th grade class. I had her in my first hour homeroom class, and she always seemed happy to be there. She was pleasant with me, and I thought comfortable enough to tell me if something was upsetting her. After about the first week of school, I noticed she was often late to my math class and repeatedly asked to use the restroom or see the nurse. I started to get suspicious, so I asked her if she was having some issues that I should be concerned with. While on the verge of tears, she told me she had stomach pains. I didn't push her during this encounter. Her requests to visit the restroom and nurse continued for another week and quickly became a disturbance to the whole class. On one of the occasions when she was returning from the restroom, I met her in the hallway because she had been gone for half the class period. When she stopped to talk to me, she was crying, and I couldn't get her to share her feelings. She only wanted the nurse. Later that day, the nurse confided in me that she thought the girl was dealing with anxiety. That got me thinking is she doing this in other classes or is it just my math class? I asked the other core teachers, and they hadn't noticed any of these particular behaviors from the student. They actually raved about her abilities in their subjects. At this point she was displaying all the signs of "math anxiety." Now that I understood what was happening with her, I took steps to help her through her anxiety such as giving extra time and gently making sure she understood concepts. We developed a positive relationship, and she actually enjoyed math class.

Math anxiety can also be communicated from teachers. Consider elementary teachers who were followed from their teacher education training to five years of experience (Gresham, 2018). All in the study experienced math anxiety. Their anxiety decreased somewhat across the 5 years, but was still severe. Here are some of their comments:

Teacher A: Ever since I was in elementary school I have hated math! Literally! I remember going home crying, not wanting to go to school, screaming at my mother for making me do my homework, stressing out over not knowing how to do it, and begging her to let me quit school. And all this by 5ᵗʰ grade! I always got sick during math class and could feel my blood pressure rise every day. This never stopped during my years in high school either. I know I had math anxiety, I know I hated math, and I know I never wanted to see it again once I graduated from high school. Now I'm trying to be a teacher and I still hate math. How will I be able to help my students if I hate it?

(p. 96)

Teacher B: I noticed so many students struggled that year because of me. I knew I had to change my attitude towards math because I set the tone for the day and it was negative. …That's changed the last few years. I think implementing the strategies I learned and seeing my students be more successful has helped ease my stress in knowing that "I can do this math stuff and yes, they can do this math stuff!" Yes, I am still overwhelmed but I try not to let my students see or sense my frustration because it causes me more stress!

(p. 96)

Teacher C: One day I was teaching a concept and literally cried in front of my kids because I didn't get it either. When I expressed my disdain towards mathematics and my students witnessed my meltdown they immediately shut down and I lost them during math lessons for weeks afterwards. I know that seeing their teacher get frustrated with the math left a long lasting if not lifelong impression on them.

(p. 97)

These comments highlight the importance of teachers having positive attitudes toward the topics they teach. While no teacher will love every topic or be equally competent at every topic, it is devastating to students' motivation if their teachers communicate fear or dislike for what they are teaching. The same teachers reported that as they learned to use manipulatives (concrete objects that are used to count and to illustrate mathematical principles like regrouping 10's) to teach and understand mathematics, their anxiety decreased and their students responded positively. Some came up with relevance comments (discussed in more detail in Chapter 6) like the following:

One student never wanted to do his work, would misbehave, and keep others from getting their work done. One day he asked me when they would see this stuff and I told him that was a good question. I asked him what time he got up in the morning, how much money he had for his lunch that day, and how much it was going to cost him for the field trip we were going on Friday? He just looked at me kind of puzzled. Then he looked at me and smiled. I was so excited and proud of myself! He is now the first one to get going on his work and wants to be involved in everything we are doing. He was struggling with multiplication and I brought in some manipulatives to help. Instead of misbehaving like he used to do, he got busy playing and trying to work the problems. I think he sees what he needs math for now.

(p. 97)

Female students who have math-anxious female teachers tend to endorse stereotypes about girls being bad at math and also experience lowered math achievement (Beilock et al., 2010). Similar research has not been done with male teachers, but it seems likely that they also can communicate stereotypes and math anxiety. This means that you, as a parent, teacher, or counselor, should guard against making comments that imply some people are good at math (or any other topic) and others are not (fixed mindset).

Background Knowledge

Students feel competent when they have knowledge of a domain. Knowledge of a domain is particularly important for reading comprehension (as described in the Introduction). That is, when a reader reads material about a familiar topic, the reader's background knowledge is activated. Someone who knows nothing about DNA or genetics is not likely to understand or be interested in CRISPR for gene editing. Someone who has relevant background knowledge is likely to be fascinated. Similarly, someone who knows nothing about the Mexican Revolution except that Pancho Villa was involved is not likely to understand or be interested in an analysis of the roles of Porfirio Diaz, Emiliano Zapata, or Venustiano Carranza. Someone who has visited Mexican battle sites and learned about the people just listed is likely to be fascinated by new information about Álvaro Obregón and Plutarco Calles. Background knowledge is related to interest such that people with high interest are likely to increase their knowledge, and people high in background knowledge are likely to be interested and even increase in interest (Alexander et al., 1995; Falk & Adelman, 2003; Linnenbrink-Garcia et al., 2012; Murphy & Alexander, 2002; Tobias, 1994; Zhang et al., 2016). That is, as people learn more about a topic, they tend to increase in interest and motivation for that topic. This means that a key aspect of instruction is helping learners generate a dense network of connected pieces of knowledge for the domain they are studying.

Deliberate Practice

Competence requires practice, but many children and youth are not motivated to practice. Practice and repetition are necessary for improving social skills, academic skills, physical therapy skills, and any other skill that is worthwhile. A six-year-old cello prodigy, Marc Yu, who had recently lost three teeth, gave advice on how to improve: "You should play Game Boy less, and you should practice more" (Hulbert, 2018, p. x). Even standup comedians must practice. The book *Mastering Stand-up* (Rosenfield, 2018) points out that good comedians practice all the time. The basketball player Ray Allen, who was the NBA career leader in three-pointers, was annoyed when people said he was a natural, as though he did not need to practice. "When people say God blessed me with a beautiful jump shot, it really pisses me off. I tell those people, 'Don't undermine the work I've put in every day.'" But kids in school, music, and sports often do not realize how much practice it takes to get good at a skill. They may not be motivated to practice or might not know how to practice. Just doing homework and playing a sport are not effective forms of practice. A role of the parent, teacher, or coach is to teach about the importance of being motivated to practice and *how* to practice.

Anders Ericsson, an expert on how to become an expert, noted that merely participating in an activity does not necessarily result in expertise or even improvement. We all know athletes, language learners, and musicians who "practice" but do not improve their skills. Ericsson and colleagues developed the notion of *deliberate practice* as an explanation for why some people consistently improve. Deliberate practice is different from mere practice. Deliberate practice refers to engaging in tasks that are specifically designed to increase competence and that have the following attributes (Ericsson, 2021; Ericsson & Pool, 2016):

1 the task has a clear goal;
2 the participant is able to practice the task alone;
3 the participant acquires objective feedback which allows modification of behavior which improves performance;
4 practice involves repetition;
5 the practice tasks are designed by instructors or coaches who individualize practice;
6 the learner engages in full concentration.

Ericsson also noted that deliberate practice may not be enjoyable. As learners gain skill through practice, their self-efficacy rises and so does their motivation.

While not all practice is deliberate practice, improvement will not occur without some kind of practice. Consider reading. Some children enter kindergarten having spent more than 1,000 hours reading with their parents. Other kindergarteners may have only ten to 20 hours (Adams, 1990). While reading with parents does not have all of the attributes of deliberate practice, it is a form of practice and does affect reading competence. Children who have been read to by their parents enter school with better prereading skills than other children and greater motivation to read.

Part of being an effective teacher, counselor, or coach, is convincing children that they need motivation to practice in order to master important skills. The practice cannot be haphazard or occasional. It needs to be frequent, with feedback, and using tasks that will actually result in improvement. It cannot be going-through-the-motions practice.

Engaging in deliberate practice and maintaining persistence require motivation. Children who become expert may have a higher level of drive to improve and a greater willingness to practice. You probably know youth who hate practicing in some domains, like the piano, but don't want to quit practicing in other domains, like their favorite hobbies, sports, or video games.

An important implication from the research on talent development is the need to convince learners that deliberate practice is required for expertise. If learners believe that talent is innate, and that people who have innate talent do not have to practice hard, they will tend to avoid effort. They will have a fixed mindset. And they will not improve as much as they could. To counter these beliefs and help all your students—whether gifted or not—to develop expertise, follow these guidelines:

1 *Provide time to practice.* If learners do not put in the time, they will not gain the skill. However, mere time is not sufficient to develop high expertise.
2 *Make sure practice is deliberate.* Assign challenging and complex tasks that require effort and mindfulness. Provide feedback so learners accurately understand what it takes to be successful. Make sure adequate materials and facilities are available. Provide tasks that learners can repeatedly practice when alone.
3 *Help learners feel motivated to engage in deliberate practice.* How to encourage feeling motivated is described throughout this book.
4 *Explain to learners the importance of deliberate practice.* Share stories of people who appear to be supremely talented, but who practiced intensely. Their practice may not have had all the attributes of deliberate practice, but they practiced more intensely and with more feedback than people who just do the activity. Sharing stories can be done through examples like the following.

Examples of Deliberate Practice

Bill Gates, co-founder of Microsoft, engaged in a lot of computer practice when he was young. When he was in 8th grade, the school that Bill Gates attended started a computer club. Gates reported, "They put three thousand dollars into a computer terminal down in this funny little room that we subsequently took control of." Gates spent many hours in that funny room. Soon a company asked if the computer club would like to test out the company's software in exchange for free computer time. In response, Gates rode a bus to the company offices and programmed many hours to earn computer time. In one seven-month period in 1971, Gates and his friends used 1,575 hours of mainframe computer time, which averages out to eight hours a day, seven days a week. "It was my obsession," Gates says of his early high school years. "I skipped athletics. I went up there at night. We were programming weekends. It would be a rare week that we wouldn't get 20 or 30 hours in" (adapted from Gladwell, 2008, pp. 50–55). Bill Gates was not so gifted that he did not need practice.

Lindsey Vonn, the retired ski racer, has more women's World Cup victories, 82, than anyone else. How did she get so good? As a child, she was mediocre at soccer, not good at figure skating, and was not even good at kickball, so it seems that she was not a natural athlete (Vigneron, 2013, Feb). As a child skier, she was called a "turtle" by her coach. However, she practiced. A lot. She said, "I got more slalom gates in than any kid in the country by, I don't know, tens of thousands" (p. 46). When she was older, she regularly took notes about her gear and her practices. Her off-season training included up to seven hours in the gym each day, six days a week. Her approach to deliberate practice paid off in victories.

Russell Thomas was an 18-year-old basketball player at Abraham Lincoln High School when it won a New York City high school championship in Madison Square Garden. During the summer offseason, he would avoid pickup games and work out instead. He would spend an hour shooting 3-pointers, sprint up and down the fourteen flights of stairs in his project building, and then shoot with one hand while sitting in a chair ten feet from the basket (Frey, 1994). He also practiced defensive footwork with a ten-pound brick in each hand. His approach to deliberate practice paid off in competence.

Your learners need to know that people who excel, like the people just described, really practiced. They were effortful and strategic. I love Bobbie Kelsey's statement when she was head women's basketball coach at the University of Wisconsin. She emphatically stated what it takes to be a great shooter:

> If people think they goin' to get it on the pillowcase, it's not going to happen. You can't nap your way to being a great shooter. And facebookin' and all these things that teenagers do. You need to put the phones down. Stop face timin'. Stop tweetin'. And *get your butt in the gym.*
>
> (Kelsey, 2016)

Your clients, students, and athletes will benefit from your careful thinking about and implementing the kinds of practice that most foster growth.

Deliberate Practice for Professionals

Access to deliberate practice is a problem for professionals like teachers and therapists who want to improve their own practice and know that improving their practice is key to fostering motivation in children and youth. Teachers and therapists only occasionally get feedback. Teachers often participate in professional development activities, but they are mostly lecture that may include small amounts of practice with feedback. This makes it difficult for teachers to consistently improve. The same pattern is true of therapists.

Expert teachers develop over time, and deliberate practice can play a role. Notice that people who seem to be born teachers were often motivated to teach their siblings or dolls when they were young, graduated to camp counselors, and so forth. They practiced a lot before they even received training. They did not "start teaching" when they got their first jobs. Deliberate practice for teachers might include participating in (not just attending) workshops, observing other teachers' classrooms, revising lesson plans based on reflection, and practicing delivery of lessons. However, feedback is critical to deliberate practice, and typical teaching practice in the US does not include critical and deep feedback. The same is true of therapists and coaches. Therapists and teachers usually practice behind closed doors. Coaches perform in public when their athletes compete, but their practices are usually behind closed doors. Feedback can be threatening, and people often avoid it precisely because it is threatening. But avoiding feedback undermines improvement just as self-handicapping undermines student improvement.

In Japan, teachers are given time to craft lessons and share ideas about how to improve lessons. A leading math teacher once attracted 1,000 observers to a public lesson (Greer, 2014). He was also featured on a television show. In China, teachers have research groups in which they practice by giving public lessons to real students in front of fellow teachers (Han & Paine, 2010). The teachers who were studied chose topics that are difficult for students to grasp. When math teachers prepared their lessons, they focused on three tasks: 1) designing mathematical tasks for students that would teach a difficult mathematical idea, 2) teaching the difficult mathematical idea, and 3) using mathematically, pedagogically appropriate language.

During the preparation phases, the Chinese teachers carefully generated lesson plans regarding exactly what they would say and what tasks they would give the students. They received feedback on the lesson plans from multiple people who could be from the same school or even schools in distant cities. They anticipated student misconceptions and had appropriate strategies prepared. They revised their lesson plans based on feedback. They tried out the lesson with students from their own school, perhaps four or five times. They revised based on reflection about their experience. They finally presented their public lesson. In the research, one teacher presented to 16 teachers and another presented to 70. They received feedback from the observers that included lengthy discussions of student responses and misconceptions. Note that observers also improved their teaching practice because of their participation. Imagine the increase in motivation learners would have if their teachers had the level of deliberate practice I have been describing. Instruction would be so much more engaging.

A school in New York City has used a similar approach in which several teachers planned a lesson together, observed each other teaching, discussed how it went, improved the lesson, and tried again. Sometimes 20 teachers observed the revised lesson and gave feedback (Kenny, 2012). A math teacher said that this form of iterative practice with reflection and feedback transformed the way he taught:

> I used to deliver information to students about mathematical formulas: some of them got it, others didn't. Now I facilitate a process where they have to do the work of discovering and understanding the concepts so deeply that they are able to devise the formulas.
>
> (p. 214)

His practice improved performance on the state proficiency test; students said the test was easier than their class work. The public lesson helps the performing teacher, *and* the observing teachers, *and* the students. It is clear that students are more motivated to learn when lessons are presented in an effective, interesting way.

Summary

- Feeling competent is a key component of motivation.
- When students' perceptions of competence are threatened, they increase self-handicapping, which refers to doing things that protect one's ego by avoiding high effort.
- Self-efficacy is a key competence concept and refers to individuals' beliefs in their ability to exert control over themselves and their environment.
- People with high efficacy tend to have high performance, use high quality strategies, overcome barriers, persist, and commit to challenging goals.
- Self-efficacy has four major influences:

  a   Mastery experience, or previous success (or lack of success).
  b   Vicarious experience, or learning from models.
  c   Persuasion, or messages from others.
  d   Physiological states such as anxiety and fatigue.

- Self-efficacy interventions use the influences on efficacy to improve learners' efficacy:

a   Foster mastery experience.
b   Provide or draw attention to models, especially peer models and coping models.
c   Tell learners that they are capable and draw attention to their previous success.
d   Structure environments to avoid negative physiological states like anxiety.
e   Use mastery modeling.

- When learners experience high anxiety, it can be useful to suggest that it means that they are learning, not that they are failing.
- When students are led to believe that a field requires brilliance, females and African Americans are less likely to pursue that field. One way to combat the belief that a field is only for certain people is to teach how even apparently brilliant people struggled in their fields.
- Math anxiety can undermine performance in math. Some interventions help reduce math anxiety. Teachers can communicate math anxiety.
- Deliberate practice refers to engaging in tasks that are specifically designed to increase competence.
- Deliberate practice has the following attributes:

a   The task has a clear goal.
b   The participant is able to practice the task alone.
c   The participant acquires objective feedback.
d   Practice involves repetition.
e   The practice tasks are designed by instructors or coaches.
f   The learner engages in full concentration.
g   Practice may not be enjoyable.

- People who have been highly successful have engaged in deliberate practice.
- Participating in deliberate practice can be difficult for professionals like teachers, therapists, and coaches.
- Rich background knowledge supports perceptions of competence and interest.

Suggestions for Further Reading

Bandura, A. (1997). *Self-efficacy: The Exercise of Control*. Freeman.
Ericsson, K. A., & Pool, R. (2016). *Peak: Secrets from the New Science of Expertise*. Mariner Books.
Usher, E. L. (2009). Sources of middle school students' self-efficacy in mathematics: A qualitative investigation. *American Educational Research Journal, 46*(1), 275–314.

Chapter 4

Do Children and Youth Feel that They Belong?

The Importance of Connection, Caring, and Relationships

Belongingness refers to feeling a connection with others, a feeling that others accept and care about you. Humans have a need to belong with others and to form meaningful interpersonal relationships (Baumeister & Leary, 1995). In school settings, belongingness, also termed relatedness, can occur 1) between adults and learners and 2) among learners. Children and youth can feel belongingness with therapists, counselors, and coaches. There is considerable evidence that when learners feel a relationship with the adults around them, they are more motivated and learn more than when they do not. When students feel their teachers like them, they tend do better in school and like school more (Wang & Eccles, 2013). Compared with students who do not have good relationships with their teachers, students with close teacher relationships are more likely to experience academic interest, academic achievement, good behavior, self-efficacy, and motivation (Fast et al., 2010; Roorda & Koomen, 2021; Roorda et al., 2011; Sakiz et al., 2012; Tosto et al., 2016; Wentzel et al., 2010). Research that followed students from kindergarten to third grade found that students whose teachers reported good relationships with them in kindergarten had better motivational attitudes in third grade, and these positive patterns predicted better achievement at the end of elementary school (Zee et al., 2021). This pattern of results means that fostering belongingness among learners is likely to enhance motivation, well-being, and achievement.

Paths to Belongingness

As you think about how to foster belongingness, it is useful to think about four different paths to belongingness (Hirsch & Clark, 2018). First, communal relationship refers to feeling close bonds with other people; this means that you would look out for them and they would look out for you. You feel that there are people to whom you could turn in times of need and that people could turn to you in their times of need. Second, general approbation refers to receiving praise or admiration from others, especially people with status. Third, group membership refers to being a member of

DOI: 10.4324/9781003046516-4

a group. The group could be a group like one's ethnic group or it could be a group that one joins like a sports team or a classroom. Fourth, minor sociability refers to briefly connecting with others through behaviors such as being pleasant, making eye contact, and smiling.

Instructors can foster all four paths to belonging.

1   They foster communal relationships when they know about learners and staff around them. They know names, hobbies, and family members. They notify learners of relevant activities, such as tryouts for the upcoming play. The ask about a family's well-being, like how the new little sister is doing.
2   They give approbation when they praise learners like commenting on specifics about an essay they wrote or their performance in a public event.
3   They foster group membership when they invite all to join the group, whether the group is a classroom, a sports team, a school, or a community.
4   They foster minor sociability when they are pleasant and welcoming in chance encounters in places such as the hallway and classroom.

Instructor-learner Relations

Instructor-learner relations are a key part of fostering learners' sense of belongingness (Bergin & Bergin, 2009; Hagenauer & Volet, 2014). Therapists and coaches are analogous to instructors. Research on instructor-learner relationships with K–12 children has consistently shown positive correlations between teacher-student relationships and student motivation and learning outcomes (Bergin & Bergin, 2009; Robinson et al., 2019).

Learners of color often feel less relatedness in formal learning settings, especially when their instructors do not look like them or when they are the only person of color in the group. Immigrant students may feel lack of relatedness due to social isolation and lack of social support. Their alienation can be exacerbated if they do not speak the local language. This means that educators may need to pay special attention to students of color and immigrant students.

Instructors can foster belongingness and relatedness by following these guidelines:

•   *Get to know each other.* Know all learners' names and encourage them to know each others' names. Have them share something about each other—interests, families, background—to foster personal connections.
•   *Be appropriately warm and welcoming.* Listen, give appropriate advice, and acknowledge learners' expressions of negative emotion. Behavior as simple as looking at people and smiling reduces their feelings of

disconnection, whereas being ignored, even by strangers, increases feelings of disconnection (Wesselmann et al., 2012).

- *Avoid microaggressions.* Microaggressions are subtle messages that communicate bias or prejudice; they are often unintentional and subconscious (Sue et al., 2007). Examples might include an instructor complimenting learners from a different background on their articulateness or treating students who do not speak English well as invisible and unimportant. Not including course material generated by people of color can communicate lack of interest in learners of color. Inform yourself about possible microaggressions and go out of your way to avoid them. The topic of microaggressions is expanded in Chapter 8.

Stacy Bess taught in an elementary classroom in a community homeless shelter in Salt Lake City. Her students came from very difficult circumstances and did not feel that they belonged to a community. She told the students that they would begin each day with a "jam session":

"We all sit together in a circle, and whatever you need to say, you can say it," I told them. "It never leaves the circle, and we get a chance to help each other solve our problems." I had found that the kids liked our jam sessions because they got to talk about anything and everything. This gave them a chance to help each other and to learn that they weren't alone in their fears and their worries. Sometimes we got horror stories—an arrest, a drug bust, a knife fight from the night before. Sometimes stories of hope—Katie's father just landed a job; Rob's sister had her new baby. The jam sessions have been more valuable to me than any college course on social issues could ever dream of being for gaining firsthand an understanding of homelessness from the people it affects the most—the children.

(Bess, 1994, p. 50)

Bess had some very tough situations, but she still tried to create bonds with children and their families. For example, a homeless mother brought her five-year-old Tucker to the classroom. Tucker looked into his new teacher's eyes and said, "I'm going to kill you." He would kick and scream when his mother left him. He frequently urinated in the classroom. Bess held Tucker and rocked him and cleaned up after his urinations. She sat on the floor and talked with Patty, Tucker's mother, and learned that Patty was a priestess in the Satanic church and Tucker was a "guardian" in the church. During art, Tucker would draw human figures and cut off the arms, legs, and heads. Tucker was taken into protective custody and his abusive father was kicked out of the shelter. Bess continued to try to build bonds with Tucker and his mother and the other children in her classroom.

It can be particularly difficult to build bonds with children who are aggressive, smelly, or unattractive. Bess described nine-year-old Dana, who acted afraid much of the time. "Because Dana wasn't cute, cuddly, or even attractive, both adults and peers found it easy to ignore her. She moped around on the sidelines of every activity, lonely and withdrawn" (Bess, 1994, p. 68). After she got Dana to look at her without fear, Bess invited her to come to class early, and Bess would brush her tangled hair and make her look "cool." They developed a rapport. Later, Bess discovered that before coming to Salt Lake, a sheriff had discovered Dana and her brother locked in windowless dirt-floored cellar with no food or water. They were being "punished" by the mother and her boyfriend. It is especially important to reach out to the children who seem less lovable.

Laura Raicu taught on the west side of Chicago. The neighborhoods experienced severe gang violence, and two students had been recently killed in gang-related shootings. She was feeling despair when another teacher asked a student what he most liked about Ms. Raicu.

> "Sometimes," he said slowly, "the only reason I come to school is because of Ms. Raicu. She's always here for me." That was all he needed to say. I held in my tears until we said our goodbyes. Then, like a waterfall, I let them run down my cheeks and chin. They were tears of pain, joy, and relief.
>
> (Raicu, 2017, p. 15)

Labeling students in positive ways can foster their prosocial behavior and kindness. When students treat each other with kindness, it increases feelings of belongingness. Wendy Keppley (2017) described when she was eight-years' old and a new girl with a horribly scarred left leg joined the class. Her name was Margaret Cooper, and Wendy and her friends immediately came up with names like Margaret Cooper Pooper and Maggot Pooper. Before the day was over, Wendy's teacher pulled her aside and said that because Wendy was a nice person and a leader in the class, it would be important for Wendy to lead the way in welcoming Margaret into the class. Wendy immediately felt guilty for participating in the behind-the-back name calling and quickly became friends with Margaret. Without the teacher's intervention, the experiences of Wendy and Margaret would have been quite different.

A key component of feeling belongingness is emotional. In a teacher training session, the trainer showed a photo of a student staring into space and then resting his head on his desk (Emdin, 2016, p. 29). The trainer asked the professional development teachers to describe the student. They described him as disinterested or unmotivated. The trainer then showed a video of the student repeatedly trying to answer a question, raising his hand, and finally calling out the answer after he was ignored. The student had an emotional reaction to being ignored that looked like lack of motivation. But he did not lack motivation. He felt rejected and ignored. The teachers did not see this in the single snap-shot photo, which is the sort of view teachers often get during classroom interaction.

Research and Theory into Practice

A review of literature (Bergin & Bergin, 2009) on teacher-student relationships provided specific guidelines based on research of what adults can do to foster a good relationship with each child. These guidelines apply to other adults like parents, coaches, and therapists:

1   Increase sensitivity and warm, positive interactions with learners. One way to increase sensitivity is to increase understanding of child development such as how emotions develop and what is normal at certain ages (like tantrums or ability to control negative emotions).
2   Be well prepared for class, therapy session, or sports practice and communicate high expectations. Help learners with their activities. Respond to their questions and concerns.
3   Provide choice whenever possible to respond to their preferences. Choice may be less important for children from collectivist cultures compared to individualist cultures (Iyengar & Lepper, 1999; Katz & Assor, 2007).
4   Avoid power assertion and coercive discipline such as making threats and using superior power to coerce compliance. Use induction instead, which involves explaining the reason for rules and the consequences, especially for others, of breaking rules. For example, when a child hits other children or takes their toys, the other children feel sad. When an athlete hogs the ball, it hurts the team.
5   Help youth be prosocial, that is, kind to and accepting of each other. Prosocial behaviors include comforting distressed peers; helping others with sports, academic work, or social problems; inviting others to join groups; apologizing when appropriate; and avoiding hurting others' feelings. Adults can undermine prosocial behavior when they punish children for helping each other, such as saying "Don't talk to other students in class. Come to me if you have a problem."

Interview: Feeling a Bond with Fellow Students

High School English Teacher at a Rural School. Seven Years of Experience

I teach acting classes in addition to English, and this past year there came a point a few weeks into the semester where my acting class of

9th-12th graders was just dragging. Many of the kids were quieter than usual, getting easily frustrated, and generally being unwilling to work with one another, which is obviously a major problem in a theater class that is built around collaboration. I'd also heard some muttered disparaging comments here and there about other people in the class. I took time the next day to address my observations and concerns, and as a class, we spent the next hour sitting in a circle on the floor of the auditorium stage discussing (and sometimes venting about) what was on everyone's mind. I learned a lot about things I could do to help make things better, and everyone else learned a lot about each other. By the end of class, I asked everyone to openly say a meaningful positive comment to someone else in the circle, one at a time until everyone had said and received one. One student stayed behind to cry for a minute or two because it had been a long time since anyone had genuinely said something nice about them and they had no idea someone saw them that positively. Several more students asked the next day if we could do that sort of thing again. After that day, the class dynamic was outstanding.

One teacher wrote that students "live for three things: recess, lunch, and sharing" (Done, 2005, p. 80). Sharing time can foster classroom relationships and belonging. However, this teacher also found that sharing in a third-grade class can involve excessive family disclosure such as what a dad says about his mother-in-law's Jell-O salad or who slept on the couch last night. One child brought in a bag for sharing time that he announced was full of ladybugs. He claimed that his uncle, a farmer, ordered ladybugs every year to put on the crops. The teacher was dubious that you can just order ladybugs, so guess what? The kid opened the bag! So be careful as you implement activities to foster belongingness.

Caring can come from school personnel who are not teachers, counselors, or administrators. An adult who experienced learning difficulties as a child reported that a custodian helped him feel cared for in his school, where he spent a lot of time in the hallway due to being sent out of class (Flink, 2014). Jim, the custodian, high fived, joked, and played chess with the fourth grader (and frequently lost the chess matches to the fourth grader). "Jim was my salvation. In fourth grade, if not for Jim, his smiles, and his chess set, I would have given up" (p. 203).

Teachers need to communicate their fondness for students because students may not notice that they are cared for. Frank McCourt (2005) told the story of Bob, a young man in his high school class who wore a double-breasted jacket that he claimed once belonged to Orson Welles. His pants were cutoffs. He did not bring paper or writing utensil to the writing class. He was in an elite New York City school and wanted to become a farmer. Six years later teacher and former student met by chance, Bob in his

Orson Welles jacket and cutoffs in January. Bob asked, "Mr. McCourt, you never liked me, did you?" (p. 240). So, Mr. McCourt told Bob that he was a joy to have in class because he drove away gloom, had good humor, and was honest and courageous. But Mr. McCourt had not communicated that fondness while Bob was a student. Six years is a long time to wait.

A teacher must know the students in order to help them feel accepted and valued. A new middle school principal was visited by her mentor, a former principal (Lopez, 2016). The mentor named some students and asked the principal about them. The principal gave an answer filled with vague generalities. The mentor said,

> Let me explain something to you. You work in an underserved community. And what's going to happen is everyone is going to tell you what these kids *can't* do. The data from the tests will say these kids aren't achieving. The media will say they can't act right. Your teachers will say they can't learn. It's much easier to say what kids are deficient in than to figure out what they're great at and work hard to build upon their abilities. So the next time I come here and ask you that question, you better have a real answer to give me.... You owe that to these children.
>
> (Lopez, 2016, p. 58)

The principal said that was one of the best pieces of advice she ever received. She took home files for the children and made notes about their strengths and weaknesses. She pieced together the whole child. She then asked her teachers about their own students, and the teachers struggled to give specifics. The principal assigned them to learn all they could about each child in order to respond to their individual needs.

Some schools provide little or no time for students to interact with each other or with teachers outside of classrooms. Students may have back-to-back classes, short intervals between classes, 30-minute lunch, no talking permitted in study halls, and long commutes to and from school. They are with other people all day but literally have only minutes in which they can casually interact with teachers and fellow students. Students need to have time to converse with each other and with teachers, administrators, and staff.

Teachers can connect with students when they go the extra mile. Caroline McKinney (2017) had a ten-year-old student, Sean, who was constantly in trouble. When she read picture books aloud to the group, he did not seem interested. However, one day she read *Heckedy Peg* by Audrey Wood with pictures by Don Wood. The story is about a mother who outwits a child-stealing witch. At the story's end, Sean called out that the ending was bad, and he could have done better. In the course of the conversation, teacher McKinney realized that Sean liked and could discuss all the books she had read. She told Sean to write down his improved ending for *Heckedy Peg*, and she would mail it to the authors, which she did. This occurred in May, and in August she tracked down Sean in another classroom to deliver the responding letter from Audrey Wood. Sean was stunned and pleased at the response that acknowledged his thoughtful suggestions and encouraged him to continue to be a creative thinker. This experience that was engineered by a teacher was a key moment for Sean and improved his attitude toward school.

Sometimes reaching out to a student, even secretly, helps motivate them. Olly Neal was a student in Arkansas who was trouble (adapted from Kristof, 2012; Taing, 2009). He shoplifted where he worked and was so difficult that he reduced his English teacher, Mrs. Grady, to tears. Another teacher said that in order to deal with students like Olly, she would practice being mean in front of a mirror. During his senior year, he cut class one day and went to the library to escape. He noticed a book with a sexy woman on the cover. He wanted to read the book, but was afraid that his friends might see him with a book and tease him. He said he wanted to be known for fighting and swearing and not for reading. He stole the book, that is, borrowed it without checking it out. The book was by Frank Yerby, a best-selling Black author. Yerby's book *The Foxes of Harrow*, a Southern historical romance, was the first novel by an African American to sell more than a million copies. Weeks later Olly snuck the book back into the library and noticed another book by Yerby. He stole that one too, and ended up reading four books by Yerby. He loved reading and went on to read Camus and other challenging authors. He went to law school and became an appellate judge in the Arkansas Court of Appeals. At his thirteenth high school reunion, he learned that Mrs. Grady, who was also the librarian, had noticed him stealing the first book. She understood why he was stealing, so she drove 70 miles to Memphis to buy another Yerby book. She did this three times, each time placing the book on the shelf where Olly would find it. Her secret caring changed Judge Neal's trajectory and vicariously influenced his daughter, who earned a PhD in genetics.

Sometimes a small gesture has a powerful impact. At the end of the elementary school year, John Buentello (2017) was disappointed that he had not connected with little Ashley, who was quiet and compliant but joyless. On an impulse, on the last day of the school year, he took a children's book he had recently bought and inscribed it for Ashley. She left with the book. Sixteen years later, he received an email:

> Hi Mr. Buentello,
>
> You were my third grade teacher. I'm all grown now, but I'll never forget when you gave me a book on the last day of school. You wrote a note on the inside. While it probably was a small gesture to you, it really meant a lot to me. At the time my life was very unstable.

Reading has always been an inspiration for me. The gift you gave me was the first book I ever owned, and I will never forget the moment you gave it to me. I just wanted you to know how thankful I am.

(p. 341)

Communication with Parents Can Foster Belongingness

Telling parents the good things that their children do can be a good way to create bonds with children and their parents. We knew a middle school teacher who would set aside time to phone parents to tell them about the *good* things that their child had done. He was popular with students and parents.

Let's see what happened with another teacher, Mr. Mali, and Caleb, a difficult 7th-grader who challenged him on a poorly written geometry quiz item. Mr. Mali told Caleb to prove his point for homework. That evening, Mr. Mali called Caleb's mother.

It was not the first time one of his teachers had ever called home—I got the sense that she was used to fielding such calls—but it was the first time anyone had ever told her anything good. I wanted her to know that the intellectual curiosity and vivacity that her son had displayed in class reminded me why I chose to teach in the first place. I told her that I loved my job because of kids like Caleb. The quality of silence on the other end of the phone told me that she was *crying*. By reaching out to her that night I had created an ally.

(Mali, 2012, p. 36)

Teacher Danny Brassell (2017) had a particularly difficult student, seven-year-old Belinda. She poked a classmate in the eye with a pencil. She called other students bad names. She fought. Brassell tried time out, which came to be called "jail." That did not work. He made Belinda clean the classroom during recess. She said she liked to clean and asked to do it every day. He made her copy text as punishment. Finally, he threatened to call her mother. Belinda gloated that her mother did not have a phone. Brassell said he would walk Belinda home and talk with her mother. That created silence. Belinda attempted to rapidly exit when the bell rang, but Brassell caught up with her. Brassell held her hand during the short walk to her house. He pondered what to say to the mother, who asked what Belinda had done this time.

"Well, I didn't come to tell you what Belinda is doing wrong. I came to tell you what she is doing right." He said that she participated in class and was always to school on time, and that he appreciated the mother's support.

He caught a glimpse in the house, which was a mess of papers, malt liquor bottles, and dog poop. Belinda's mother suddenly paid careful attention, beamed, and listened as Brassell listed additional positive attributes. The next day, Belinda gave his legs a hug and said he was the best teacher.

In another situation, a principal had a student, Antonne, whose father had been shot in front of him (Lopez, 2016). The father survived, but Antonne was traumatized and misbehaved, especially toward authority. The principal called the mother in to talk about Antonne's misbehavior. The mother asked if she were going to be lectured about how to raise her child. Lopez said no, that Antonne had great potential, and that she was sorry the system had failed Antonne. The mother said that no one had previously said anything good about her Antonne. This conversation put them on a productive track.

Caring

Youth feel more closeness to teachers, counselors, and therapists when they feel cared for, and they are more are motivated to change. One high school student reported that she believed her chemistry teacher cared about her "Because he has actually talked to me and we've had conversations other than about school. We've had conversations as friends and not just teacher-student" (Cooper & Miness, 2014, p. 280).

Table 4.1 lists what students say about teachers whom they perceive as caring and teachers they perceive as noncaring. Note that the comments affirm attention directed toward students as individuals as well as a commitment to effectively teaching the entire group. The students' emphasis that teachers demonstrate caring when they teach effectively is noteworthy. Caring is not just being nice and asking students how they are doing; it is also teaching effectively. This same pattern should apply to therapists and

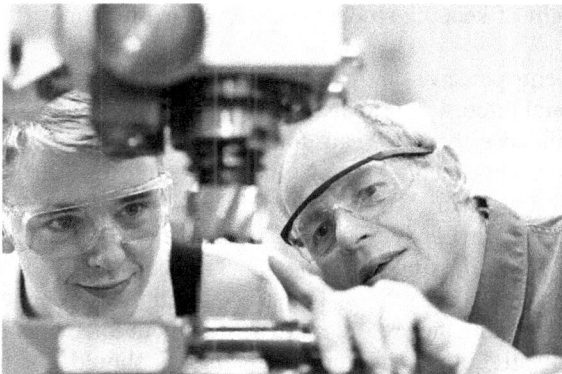

Table 4.1 Student descriptions of caring and noncaring teachers

Caring teacher behavior	*Noncaring teacher behavior*
Helps each student academically. Asks if I need help. Calls on me. Makes sure I understand.	Doesn't explain things or answer questions. Doesn't try to help.
Makes special effort. Teaches in a special way. Makes class interesting.	Gets off task. Teaches while students aren't paying attention. Boring.
Talks to me. Pays attention. Listens. Asks questions. Asks what's wrong	Screams. Yells. Ignores. Interrupts.
Knows my name.	Forgets my name.
Compliments and encourages. Checks work. Tells me when I do a good job. Praises me.	Embarrasses, insults, or picks on students. Doesn't correct work.
Trusts me, tells the truth, and keeps promises. Respects students. Avoids hurting students' feelings.	Gossips about students. Reveals private conversations with students.
They keep us safe. If there is a fire, we go outside. Goes on the roof to get balls down.	Does not call on me when I have my hand up.
Shares life experiences and stuff with us.	Doesn't ask why I'm sad. Doesn't care if I do something wrong
Greets us coming off the bus even when it is cold outside.	Sends me to the office. Gives bad grades.

Adapted from Cooper & Miness (2014), Jeffrey et al.(2013), Mirón & Lauria (1998), and Wentzel (1997).

counselors; that is, youth believe that therapists and counselors care if they provide effective interventions. In addition, in a set of interviews with elementary teachers and students, students reported that they felt cared for when they thought teachers kept them safe; the teachers had not previously thought of keeping students safe as an expression of caring (Jeffrey et al., 2013).

When students perceive that teachers care in a personal sense (our teacher takes a personal interest in us, cares how we feel, and listens to us), it boosts students' confidence that they can do academic work (efficacy), which supports their academic achievement. One study of over 1000 children that demonstrated this pattern was done with Spanish-dominant English learners in elementary school (Lewis et al., 2012). Non-English-speaking children are often cut off from classroom belongingness because they don't speak the dominant language of the school. The study found that teacher caring tended to raise student math efficacy and math achievement for English learners *and* for English fluent Latinx children. Interventions should not focus just on curriculum and content learning. Relationships affect content learning. Teacher caring boosts academic confidence which boosts achievement.

An example of high school caring shows how a caring teacher can influence student engagement. Ray, a student, was using drugs, in trouble with police, fighting, and hostile to teachers (Cooper & Miness, 2014). In Mr. Knowles' class, however, he paid attention and was respectful, so much so that other students noticed. A fellow student reported,

> [Ray is] not very good outside of school. I know he gets in a lot of trouble. His family used to be friends with my family. And I know he's into a bunch of bad things and stuff, and I noticed like one day—it was towards the beginning of the year–he was actually paying attention in class, which is weird. I mean sometimes he'll still sleep in there, but he's not rude to Mr. Knowles like he is with most other teachers— like he'll back talk. But I think it's a respect thing that Mr. Knowles gives.
>
> (p. 279)

A researcher noted that when Ray was asleep in the back of the class, Mr. Knowles walked back and whispered to him. Ray sat up. Knowles told the researcher after class that Ray worked nights from 11 pm to 4 am to help pay the family's rent. Mr. Knowles had detailed knowledge of Ray's situation and was supportive and understanding of Ray despite his sleeping in class.

In contrast, in a school that was rife with violence and climate problems, a student said that teachers did not care and used as evidence a student who could not read:

> I know a boy that's graduating right now that can't read. And you know, they not helping him by you know letting him go. It's gon' be hard for him to get a job. He's not going to be able to take care of his self. I mean, I feel like they only care about [themselves] because, if they cared about the students, they wouldn't put up with half the stuff that they do with them.
>
> (Mirón & Lauria, 1998, p. 201)

It is important to note that some students do not want to reveal themselves to teachers (Cooper & Miness, 2014). They feel that the teacher-student relationship is temporary and not part of their social or familial circle. For example, one student said, "I don't really feel comfortable talking about myself to my teachers, cause it's just for a year. They're not like my friends. They're not going to be with me for the rest of my life" (p. 280). Another said, "I don't like that whole teacher-student bond thing. There's a part where if it's too close, it's weird" (p. 281). The overall message is that your students are more likely to flourish if you have a caring, belonging rapport with them, but some might not need a relationship with their teacher.

Case 4.1

A study of student defiance was conducted at an urban high school in a mid-size city in the US (Gregory & Weinstein, 2008). Thirty African American students who received at least one defiance-related referral in one school year participated. The study found that students behaved quite differently for a liked teacher compared to the teacher who reported defiance (the referring teacher). Students reported being more rule-breaking and defiant in the referring teacher's classroom than in the liked teacher's classroom. Referring teachers perceived more defiant behavior than did the liked teachers. Students perceived more caring from, trust in, and obligation to cooperate with the liked teachers than the referring teachers. Students viewed teachers as more trustworthy if they saw the teachers as caring and academically demanding. What concepts help explain this pattern of results? How might autonomy, belongingness, and caring be relevant?

Adolescents and the Peer Group

During adolescence, youth are particularly attuned to what their peers think about them, which affects their motivation. Their drive for belongingness can have negative or positive effects. From the elementary years to age 18, youth spend increasing amounts of time with their peers (Lam et al., 2014). The peak of their time spent with same-sex peers is about age 14. As they are spending more time with peers, they are increasingly influenced by what their peers think. In one study, teens rated the risk of moderately risky behavior like riding a bicycle without a helmet, driving without a seatbelt, and drinking more than three alcoholic drinks (Knoll et al., 2017). After seeing bogus ratings by other adults or teens, they re-rated. Teens were more influenced by other teens than by adults. A review of research found that adolescents are more likely to take health and legal risks if they are with peers who value those activities than when they are alone; relevant risks include reckless behavior, dangerous driving, and experimenting with drugs, alcohol, and cigarettes (Tomova et al., 2021). At the same time, they are less likely to take social risks that might bring criticism or teasing from their peers. They have a high level of fear of being socially excluded by their peers. Note that this fear of exclusion can generate positive motivation when the peers exhibit prosocial behaviors like helping others, giving generous charitable donations, and volunteering. However, motivation to belong can have negative effects when peers exhibit negative attitudes toward learning, school, and prosocial behavior.

When teachers, parents, and other educators work with youth, it is important to be aware of the power of the peer group. While there is a stereotype that peer pressure is nearly always negative and pushes youth to do drugs, use alcohol, and drive recklessly, in fact peer pressure can be negative or positive. Youth can experience pressure from their peers to have good grades, treat others well, avoid trashy media, and share with others. Pressure for good grades can be positive, but such pressure can also be excessive and create debilitating anxiety. Nevertheless, attempts to tell youth to ignore peer norms are likely to be futile. Attempts to create motivating environments need to take into account peer norms for specific behaviors in the local peer groups. There can be peer norms for what sports to join, how to treat other ethnic groups, whether and when to use profanity, how to treat the physical environment (e.g., littering vs picking up trash), whether to use alcohol and tobacco, how to treat parents, how to treat teachers, etc. While it might be futile in the short term to push against peer norms, a long-term project could attempt to bend peer norms in more academic, prosocial, and productive directions.

Summary

- Belongingness refers to feeling a connection with others, a feeling that others accept and care about you. Humans have a need to belong with others and to form meaningful interpersonal relationships.
- There are different paths to belongingness.
- Instructor/therapist/coach relations with learners and clients are key to fostering belongingness. Adults can foster a good relationship with each child if they do the following:

  a Increase sensitivity and warm, positive interactions with learners.
  b Be well prepared for class, therapy session, or sports practice and communicate high expectations.
  c Provide choice when possible.
  d Avoid power assertion and coercive discipline such as making threats.
  e Help youth be prosocial, that is, kind to and accepting of each other.

- Communication with parents can foster belongingness.
- Caring fosters belongingness.
- Youth perceive care when adults

  a Teach effectively and help each learner to learn; teach in a special way.
  b Compliment, encourage, and praise.
  c Respect learners, tell the truth, and keep promises.

- During adolescence, youth are particularly attuned to what their peers think about them, which affects their motivation. This can have negative or positive effects.

Suggestions for Further Reading

Baumeister, R. F., & Leary, M. R. (1995). The need to belong: Desire for interpersonal attachments as a fundamental human motivation. *Psychological Bulletin, 117*, 497–529.

Bergin, C. (2018). *Designing a Prosocial Classroom: Fostering Collaboration in Students from pre-K–12 with the Curriculum You Already Use.* Norton.

Bergin, C., & Bergin, D. A. (2009). Attachment in the classroom. *Educational Psychology Review, 21*, 141–170.

Noddings, N. (1992). *The Challenge to Care in Schools: An Alternative Approach to Education.* Teachers College Press.

Chapter 5

Do Children and Youth Feel that They Have Autonomy?

The Importance of Feeling that Behavior is Freely Chosen for Well-Being and Motivation

Autonomy is a key concept in self-determination theory and refers to feeling that you are the source of your behavior and that your behavior is freely chosen (Deci & Ryan, 2002). You act based on your interests and values. You feel that the causes of your behavior come from you. You might be influenced by other people, events, or pressures, but you freely choose to go along with them rather than feeling that you are being forced to comply with them. Self-determination theory emphasizes the importance of autonomy for human well-being and motivation.

Even though autonomy is recognized as facilitating motivation and well-being, people in charge, such as teachers, parents, and supervisors, tend to feel pressure to control others.

They may think that because they are supposed to be in charge, they ought to be telling others what to do. They may tell learners or subordinates to think, feel, or behave in ways that they specify. They remove autonomy and self-determination. What can they do to support autonomy?

Supporting Autonomy

Behaviors that support autonomy include the following (Reeve, 2009; Stefanou et al., 2004; Turner et al., 2011):

- try to see things from learners' perspectives and acknowledge their perspectives.
- welcome learners' thoughts, feelings, and actions.
- nurture learners' inner motivational impulses.
- provide explanations and reasons.
- avoid controlling language like "you ought" or "you should".
- display patience.
- acknowledge and accept expressions of negative emotions.
- ask questions and don't answer them—wait for learners or clients to answer.
- encourage questions.

DOI: 10.4324/9781003046516-5

- structure instruction so that it facilitates collaboration.
- have learners speak to each other instead of to the teacher.
- encourage learners and clients to problem solve on their own.
- avoid penalizing mistakes—encourage learners to learn from mistakes.
- structure learning so that learners can pursue their own interests as much as possible.
- make learning interesting—learners would not autonomously choose to do boring things.

Start with the premise that teachers should attempt to take the students' perspective (Reeve & Cheon, 2021). Teachers can start by imagining how students might perceive instruction and assignments. However, they need more concrete data, which they can acquire by informally asking students what they think about the learning material. Teachers need to listen carefully and not just seek confirmation of their own beliefs.

In order to gather data, teachers can solicit "exit slips" in which students take the last few minutes of class or of a lesson to write their thoughts about the day's instruction, current assignments, and what they would prefer for future instruction. The exit slips can be generated on paper or a computer system. Exit slips would usually be anonymous. Teachers can provide specific prompts for exit slips (e.g., What did you think of the demonstration in today's lesson? Which concepts should be on the upcoming quiz/ exam? What were weak elements of the session we just had?) or they can be a general query about students' thoughts.

In addition to taking the students' perspective, support students' intrinsic motivation. One way to do this is to invite students to pursue their individual interests. In the next chapter, I will say more about interest. Here, suffice it to say that when students are pursuing their own interests, they are acting with autonomy. Who would autonomously choose to pursue uninteresting activities? While the curriculum will not allow complete choice of activities, instructional leaders can provide some choice. For example, in a lesson on mammals, students could choose which mammal to write about. In a lesson about WWII, students could choose a country, battle, or world leader to examine. In a physical therapy session, clients could choose between exercises or the order in which to do them (if order does not matter). However, teachers and therapists need to be careful that learners do not choose options that allow them to avoid practicing the target concepts or behaviors.

In order to support autonomy, teachers should *provide explanatory rationales* in which they explain the value and relevance (see Chapter 6 on relevance) of the learning (Reeve & Cheon, 2021). It is best to avoid merely stating that the learning is necessary for going on to the next class, though that could be mentioned. An instructor or therapist could say that others have found the learning useful and then go on to say how or why it was useful. Chapter 6 will give ideas about how to argue for usefulness. In addition to rationales, instructors and therapists should *acknowledge and accept negative feelings* among the learners. Learners may feel bored, overburdened, anxious, or fearful. The instructor should not dismiss genuine emotions, but should acknowledge that learners feel what they feel. This is related to taking the learners' perspectives, of course.

To support autonomy, instructors can use invitational language like "you might consider," "another way to think about it is," or "why do you think that happened?"

Finally, they should demonstrate patience. Instructors and therapists are often under pressure to cover material, improve test scores, and see as many clients as possible. This can cause them to be anxious to push forward and to push learners and clients to act faster. Pushing learners can cause them to shut down and terminate mental and physical engagement. Patience can allow learners figurative space and literal time to collect their thoughts, respond to tasks, and work at their own pace.

Stefanou and colleagues (2004) contrasted low and high autonomy supportive 5th and 6th grade mathematics teaching. In a low autonomy support lesson, classroom activity was directed by the teacher. The teacher began by reviewing metric measurement conversions on projected images. The students copied notes, and the teacher reminded the students what to write on their study sheet. She then gave an example of how to convert from centimeters to meters. In contrast, in a high autonomy support lesson, the students influenced the lesson and how they approached it. The teacher invited students to work alone or with peers. A student asked to change a number in the equation problem that had been posed, and the teacher agreed. The teacher gave students plenty of time to think and required students to support their claims. She encouraged them to learn from their mistakes. She asked them to describe how they were thinking about problems, which sometimes caused them to reevaluate their thinking. The autonomy supportive teachers in the study did not just provide choice. In fact, there was little choice of instructional activities or classroom setting. A key factor was that the autonomy supportive teachers encouraged independent thinking, pushed for deeper thinking, and did not just give the answers.

Undermining Autonomy

Teachers and instruction leaders may have controlling approaches that undermine autonomy (Reeve, 2009). Instructors are controlling when they do the following: pressure learners to adopt the instructor's views; intrude into learners' thoughts; use punitive if-then clauses (e.g., if you do x, then this bad thing will happen); and pressure learners to think, feel, or behave in ways that the adults specify. The use of incentives and rewards is usually controlling—why else would instructors use them? Instructors use psychological control, which also undermines autonomy, when they impose feelings of guilt or shame (e.g., you should be more like your brother), threaten to withdraw approval (I don't like you when you rile up the classroom), and encourage perfection. These are things to avoid.

Teacher behaviors that undermine autonomy include the following (Assor et al., 2005; Assor et al., 2002; Reeve, 2009):

- Force students work at a specified pace.
- Only allow opinions that fit the teacher's views.
- Give boring tasks.
- Demand compliance without providing reasons.
- Tell students what they "ought" to think, feel, or do.
- Reject students when they express negative feelings.
- Show impatience when students are slow to respond.
- Squelch student questions.
- Penalize mistakes.

Many teachers have an extrinsic theory of motivation. That is, they believe that in order to motivate students to learn and do schoolwork, someone must influence them through rewards and threats. That is why so many classrooms have systems of points, demerits, red light/green light, check marks, etc. to indicate when a student is in or out of compliance. For example, a teacher controlled her classroom by giving points or removing points for every classroom behavior. Rewards included viewing movies with popcorn for extra good behavior. She said, "I run just about everything on a token economy. Regardless of what students are doing, they always earn or lose points. I want them to be prepared for what it's like in the real world" (Sullo, 2009, p. 27).

When an interviewer asked the teacher's students what they thought, they were enthusiastic about the rewards. The interviewer asked one student what was her favorite subject? She said math because you could earn the most points in math. It was more difficult to earn points in language arts, and there were no points for art, music, or gym. When pressed about liking math, she seemed confused about whether she really liked math or just did math for the points. She said that points gave a reason to work hard and learn. The teacher even gave extra points for doing the interview. The interviewer pointed out that the students were motivated, but they were motivated to watch a movie, eat popcorn, and earn their way out of doing homework. Neither the students or the teacher mentioned the value of learning for the sake of becoming a learned person or because there is value in mathematics. There was no valuing of becoming a learned person or of learning for the sake of learning.

One problem with extrinsic motivators is that they mostly work when they are present, but when they are gone, the motivation is gone. How many teachers and therapists have used a treasure box or system of token reinforcement to shape children's behavior? They might say, "If you help clean up, you can

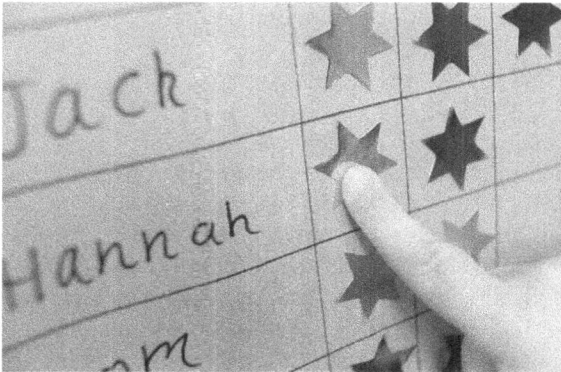

choose something out of the treasure box." When the treasures run out, the motivation goes down. In the case of trading tokens for prizes, when the attractive prizes run out, the motivation goes down—"I don't want stickers! I want candy! There's no candy left. I won't do it."

On the other hand, extrinsic motivators cannot harm intrinsic motivation if there is none. If extrinsic motivators encourage learners to develop competence, to be with other people who enjoy an activity, and to develop interest, they may develop their own intrinsic motivation for the activity. For example, people who "want" to exercise but hate it can benefit from extrinsic rewards that get them moving As they develop strength and perhaps work out with people they like, they may develop feelings of interest and enjoyment for exercise and continue even when the rewards run out.

Sometimes people in charge feel that they must crack down on subordinates, employees, and students and reduce their autonomy in order to motivate them. Managed care programs attempt to control medical care workers by incentivizing them for certain behaviors. Teachers crack down on students. For example, teacher Jennie Ivey quit accepting excuses for missing homework other than a verifiable death in the family. She was tired of the excuses. However, she reconsidered when she had a student say, "It's just that… well my dad moved out, and my mom waits tables at night, so I have to take care of my little brothers. Sometimes they cry a lot, and it makes it hard to concentrate" (p. 70). Ivey began to give the students more support for their work and focused less on cracking down. She heard additional reasons for students missing work such as

- The power company cut off our lights because my dad couldn't pay the bill.
- We had to go get my sister out of jail again.

- My mom's boyfriend locked me out of the house, so I spent the night in the car.
- My dad says schoolwork is just a waste of time.

(p. 70)

She was convinced that support was better than strict rules.

Learners will go to great lengths to resist being controlled. It is a little like whack-a-mole. When you pound down on one misbehavior, another may pop up. For example, 7th grade student Colin resented his teacher's attempts to control students. The teacher was very precise in her expectations, and she did not allow any deviation. In an interview, Colin said that he would do what the teacher said in order to preserve his grade. He said,

> Ms. Lugo has everything figured out in terms of points and value. This Civil War project counts a lot. It would be dumb not to give her what she wants in this case. But other times I blow things off and take the zero, if it's not worth that many points…. It's fun because I just like doing what I want to do and I know it drives her crazy! From the time I get up until I go to bed every day, I have people telling me what I 'have to' do. When I can do what I want without risking failure, that's pretty awesome.
> (Sullo, 2009, pp. 18–19)

Colin complies when the stakes are high, but asserts his own control and autonomy when he can.

Former teacher Frank McCourt (2005) told of a Korean American student in New York City who said that he hated his father, who had immigrated from Korea and ran a grocery store. The father made Ken, the student, take piano lessons and practice piano even though the family did not (yet) have a piano! He had to earn Eagle Scout and advance belt by belt in martial arts. He had little autonomy, and when it came time to attend college he refused to apply to Harvard or MIT, the places his father demanded, and he attended Stanford in California. He wanted to get as far from his father as possible. His mother wrote to say that he should not come home for Christmas if he had less than straight As. He said that was fine because he did not want to come home. However, at Stanford, a professor told Ken about the professor's own "son-of-a-bitch" father who survived Auschwitz and raised two kids while running a deli in Santa Barbara. The two discussed their fathers and that their fathers' desire to control their sons came from a desire to push them forward, not to harm them. The lack of autonomy felt aversive, but Ken decided to go home for Christmas and buy a tie for his father and flowers for his mother. Ken's father cared for his son (as did the professor's), but when he attempted to control Ken excessively, he lost the son's obedience and affection. There are costs to asserting control over another person.

Research and Theory into Practice

What are the effects of praise on motivation, and especially intrinsic motivation? A major review of research found that it depends (Henderlong & Lepper, 2002). Some praise can undermine intrinsic motivation and increase feelings of being controlled. Consider a coach who comments, "I am glad to see that you are doing what I told you to do." Such a comment may superficially sound like praise, but sounds to the praised like an attempt to control and could undermine motivation to listen to the coach. When praise is given for very easy tasks, it can communicate low ability— "This is so easy. Why would she praise me unless she thinks I am bad at this?" Youth who believe they have low ability tend to have low motivation. Effects of praise can vary by age. Young children, below the age of seven or so, tend to take praise literally. As they grow older, children assess the intent of praise. They may wonder if the praiser is trying to control or flatter or mislead, which can undermine motivation. The praised may ask, "Why is he saying I am so great at this task when I know I am not?" Older children will listen for sincerity and believe praise that seems sincere but discount insincere praise. Praise can be useful for communicating information, like "You did a very nice job of doing what we agreed you would do during our last therapy session." Effective praise in this situation would go on to name the specific things that were agreed upon. In summary, use sincere praise to create bonds and to communicate information about areas of competence. Avoid insincere praise that undermines your relationship. Avoid controlling praise that undermines autonomy.

Intrinsic Motivation and Autonomy

A key insight of self-determination theory is that learners can pursue tasks because they choose to, that is, autonomously, but without being intrinsically motivated. Recall from the introduction that intrinsic motivation refers to the desire to pursue an activity for its own sake, not for external reasons. Athletes may be intrinsically motivated to play a sport and to be in games, but few are intrinsically motivated for the lung-busting sprints and boring repetitions. Students may be intrinsically motivated to spend time with friends at school, but few are intrinsically motivated to sit in boring classes or answer difficult questions in class. Self-determination theory points out that even though students may not be intrinsically motivated, they can choose to engage in activities because of their autonomous decision. Even though they are not intrinsically motivated for an activity, they do not feel controlled, and their motivation is a higher quality than when they feel externally controlled. They might choose to be on a sports team in order to be with friends or to improve their fitness, not because they love the sport. They might choose to work at a fast food restaurant to earn money for a car, not because they love working in the fast food industry.

There is a continuum of extrinsic motivation that starts with behavior that is completely externally controlled with threats of punishment and promise of rewards. Then there are a series of levels of extrinsic motivation that become closer to intrinsic motivation but without being intrinsically motivated. The level that is closest to intrinsic motivation is termed *integrated regulation* (Ryan & Deci, 2020). It is autonomous because the learner chooses to do the tasks or behaviors; in addition, the learner identifies with the value of the activity and believes that the behavior fits with their own interests and values. While intrinsic motivation tends to lead to the highest quality of behavior and performance, research has shown that autonomous forms of motivation foster positive outcomes and high learner effort. This means that teachers, parents, therapists, and coaches should support learners' autonomy to pursue activities. As described above, this means taking learners' perspectives; encouraging learners to take ownership of their learning; providing interesting tasks; supporting choice; and giving rationales for learning.

Supporting autonomy should not be confused with giving learners freedom to do whatever they want. Research shows that learners benefit from structured environments, which means that teachers, therapists, parents, and coaches should, perhaps with learner input, establish goals, structure practice, give directions, communicate expectations, and provide rules (Reeve, 2009). It is important not to equate structure with control; they are different. An environment can provide structure in an autonomy-supportive manner or in a controlling manner. For example, an instructor can give a deadline (structure) just before Thanksgiving for an assignment and explain that the deadline will allow learners to relax over the holiday (rationale) and will give the instructor time to grade the assignment (more rationale). This is structured and autonomy supportive. In contrast, an instructor can give the same deadline (same level of structure) and say that is what the course deadlines are, there is no negotiation, and each day late will result in a drop of one grade. This approach feels controlling to learners. Furthermore, an instructor can say it would be nice if assignments were handed in before Thanksgiving but the deadline is flexible and students should hand in the assignment at least before December. This approach lacks structure and has the appearance of autonomy support but is too lax for most students.

Because choice is a key method of supporting autonomy, it is the next topic.

Choice

One way to support autonomy is with choice. When learners have choice, they can use their own interests and desires to select topics and activities.

Even relatively trivial choices have been shown to boost motivation and learning, such as which icon to use in a computer game that taught arithmetic procedures (Cordova & Lepper, 1996). Other choices that teachers might present to students include who to work with, what materials to use, what topic to pursue, what approach to use, how long to take, where to work, how to report results, and so forth. A meta-analysis found that in general, providing choice increases intrinsic motivation (Patall et al., 2008).

A study in high school science classrooms found that choice was particularly important for students who reported low interest; when students were highly interested, providing choice did not make much difference (Beymer et al., 2020). They also found that when students could choose with whom to work, they reported more positive emotions.

Physical therapists can ask clients what activities they want to pursue and what exercises they most enjoyed (or least disliked) prior to an injury. Then the therapist can create a plan for exercises that fit the client's preferences while still fostering physical rehabilitation.

Nancy Atwell, middle school teacher and winner of the $1 million Global Teacher Prize, wrote "In my 40-year career as a middle school English teacher, the simplest and most powerful innovation was to give my students *time* and *choice* as writers and readers" (Atwell, 2015). The author Sandra Cisneros (2015) wrote, "I don't think we can make children read anything they don't want to read, do you? True reading comes from pleasure, not obligation. When obliged to read something that doesn't speak to you, you'll ultimately forget it" (p. 310).

Active Learning

If you are familiar with different approaches to instruction, you will notice that the styles of teaching that most obviously support autonomy have labels such as inquiry teaching, project-based learning, discovery learning, problem-based learning, social constructivism, constructivism, active learning, and others. These approaches vary in their emphases, but all attempt to make students active in their thinking, less dependent on the teacher, and more dependent on their own thinking and problem solving. The students solve the problems instead of the teacher demonstrating how to solve problems. They tend to give students considerable choice.

These approaches support autonomy and motivation by putting students more in charge of their learning than more directed and didactic approaches. These approaches often use group work, which supports desire for belongingness. The approaches provide interesting, engaging activities that are active rather than passively sitting and listening. In order to foster autonomy and active learning, one teacher told his 9th grade students that they would become literary language detectives for the day (Sullo, 2009). He divided them into groups of three, gave each group the same set of five sonnets, and asked them to generate a definition of sonnet that sounded like it was from a dictionary. The students did not sit and listen; they had to figure out sonnet attributes on their own. The students were highly engaged. There was structure and independent thinking.

While these sorts of approaches can be powerful and are endorsed by various professional organizations, they do have downsides, such as they do not necessarily raise achievement (Lee & Anderson, 2013; Zhang, 2016). There are many videos that show students engaged in powerful learning with much back-and-forth discussion and active learning. However, if you look closely, you will likely notice some students gazing off at the wall or sitting stony-eyed. This means that autonomy-supportive instruction will not engage every student every time; it is not magic. When students propose incorrect answers, other students might roll their eyes or criticize even though they are not supposed to. This means that the teacher must train students to inhibit their criticizing impulses and encourage each other to take risks by making their thinking public.

A 2nd grade classroom illustrates student behavior in a constructivist classroom (Kamii, 1989). The teacher posed an arithmetic question: 19 + 13. One child said the answer was 26, and other students called out *"Agree!"* and *"Disagree!"* When the students defended their answers, most seemed to understand the answer and moved on. However, a few teased their incorrect classmates, and some who gave the wrong answer were embarrassed. Reliance upon student discussion is key for inquiry teaching, but how do students feel about it? Even if the atmosphere is supportive, some students will be embarrassed as least some of the time. According to a 5th-grader:

> [I]t can get sort of embarrassing at times, because like … you say something and everybody will raise their hand and want to say something different or they all disagree with you. And it makes you sort of feel like you want to crawl into a hole and die.
>
> (Lampert et al., 1996, p. 742)

Effective teaching requires engaging each student and training students to support each other, not teasing those who give incorrect answers. Learners will not engage in the kind of classroom discussion that makes active teaching motivating if they think they will look stupid. Teachers must work hard to provide a supportive environment. Teachers should avoid cracking up when students give completely wrong responses; instead, they should try to figure out where the reasoning went wrong. They also need to train students to discuss respectfully.

In active learning, students often work as a whole class or in groups so that they will be confronted with different views. Each group has students with different levels of ability so that all have to explain to others; having to explain is key to constructing personal understanding. The less advanced are challenged to understand thinking a bit above their own. However, you cannot assume that just because learners are discussing subject matter, they are learning; even if they are on-task, their conversations may not lead to understanding. Good inquiry teaching requires careful teaching, scaffolding, and monitoring.

Psychological Control

One way that people try to control others and "motivate" them is through *psychological control*. Psychological control refers to attempting to control another person by creating anxiety and guilt; it is a manipulative form of influence that undermines autonomy and can involve love withdrawal (e.g., if you don't do what I say, I won't love you anymore), lack of respect for the individual's identity, and intrusion into the person's thoughts and feelings (you should think and feel the way I tell you to). Research on the use of psychological control by parents shows negative effects such as depression, anxiety, lack of self-confidence, delinquency, antisocial behavior, and academic problems (Scharf & Goldner, 2018). Psychological control is marked by behaviors such the following (Barber et al., 2012):

- ridiculing (you are stupid, useless, selfish).
- embarrassing in public (yelling at a child in front of friends).
- invalidating (not asking why a child did something, correcting the child's point of view).
- violation of privacy (looking at their things without permission).
- guilting (saying the child is ungrateful or that if the child really cared about the parent/ teacher/ coach they would not cause him or her to worry; saying "you should be grateful for the education I am giving you"; saying "you ought to know this because we learned it last week").
- excessive expectations (nothing is good enough).
- comparing to others (compare child's level of anxiety with someone else).
- ignoring (walking away or not permitting child to speak).

While teachers and coaches are not parents, they often use similar strategies in attempts to motivate students. A study of youth ages 11–14 years found that learners who perceived their teachers to be psychologically controlling tended to report lack of autonomy and choice. Their teachers reported that the students were more likely to talk, make noise, and daydream. Instructional leaders, parents, coaches, and therapists should avoid using psychological control with their learners and clients.

Case 5.1

A longitudinal study followed 184 youth from age 13 to 32. Youth reported their perceptions of their parents' psychological control at age 13. Researchers observed their interaction with their romantic partner (if they had one) at age 27. The study found that youth whose parents used psychological control were in observably less supportive relationships at age 27, were less likely to be in a relationship or dating by age 32, and completed fewer years of schooling (Loeb et al., 2021). Use concepts from the book to examine why psychological control and controlling parenting might be related to negative outcomes in romantic relationships and education. How might your thoughts be relevant to other situations like classrooms, counseling, and varied forms of therapy?

Interview: Psychological Control and Discipline

Elementary Special Education Teacher at an Urban Elementary School. Two Years of Experience

I once observed a 3rd grader that was verbally harassing another student on the playground. As I was walking my students back inside, I was so caught off guard and bothered that nothing was being done about the verbal harassment that I stopped and tried talking to the student. He was avoiding my conversation at all costs, walking away and calling me mean names like bitch-ass and loser. I had to get back to my students, so I radioed the principal to help. And the discipline I saw was opposite of my experience as a kid in school. The principal just walked beside him, giving him space, and complimented him on his shoes. This interested the student enough to stand still and talk about what he was frustrated about. I was amazed! My experience with discipline in school was psychological control, where adults manipulate a child's behavior by trying to make them feel guilty or saying that they are not good people. The children at my childhood school were disciplined with remarks about potential failure. There was harsh criticism and threats that if they did not behave, they would not move on to the next grade level or be a "successful" student. This was a real threat because most of the parents of the students that attended my private school were very successful around our community. I believe that the authoritarian teaching style I received in school and at home did not foster self-control. I lived mostly in fear of discipline and punishment. I did not feel warmth from teachers or my father. My mother was a warm, authoritative parent, but she got trumped by my father's authoritarian style of parenting. Once I got older, I lacked self-confidence and began misbehaving and sneaking around when the pressure was off.

When I was in high school, we all had iPhones and were very sneaky about texting each other. We would get fined by the school if we were caught. The first offense was $25, second was $50, third was $75 and fourth would be a detention. The worst case ever would be getting caught for the fourth time on a Friday because you had to serve your detention before receiving it back, and most of the time you would lose your phone for the weekend. The thing about this power assertion is that it never worked. Time and time again, the punishment was worth the crime, especially in cases where the student got to skip out on school to serve their detention.

Summary

- Autonomy refers to feeling that you are the source of your behavior and that your behavior is freely chosen. Motivation is fostered by perceptions of autonomy.
- Behaviors that support autonomy include trying to see from learners' perspectives, providing explanation, avoiding controlling language, displaying patience, encouraging questions, accepting mistakes, making participation interesting.
- Behaviors that undermine autonomy include forcing learners to work at a specified pace, only allowing the adult's perspective, demanding compliance without reasons, penalizing mistakes.
- Many adults hold an extrinsic theory of motivation that emphasizes rewards and threats. These are less effective in the long term.
- Behavior that is self-determined but not intrinsically motivated tends to be higher quality than behavior that is externally controlled.
- Supporting autonomy does not mean total freedom. Learners benefit from structure.
- Providing choice supports autonomy.
- Active learning supports autonomy and is more motivating for learners but needs to be carefully implemented.
- Psychological control refers to attempting to control another person by creating anxiety and guilt; it is a manipulative form of influence that undermines autonomy and healthy motivation.

Suggestions for Further Reading

Grolnick, W. S. (2003). *The Psychology of Parental Control: How Well-Meant Parenting Backfires.* Lawrence Erlbaum.

Reeve, J., & Cheon, S. H. (2021). Autonomy-supportive teaching: Its malleability, benefits, and potential to improve educational practice. *Educational Psychologist, 56*(1), 54–77.

Ryan, R. M., & Deci, E. L. (2020). Intrinsic and extrinsic motivation from a self-determination theory perspective: Definitions, theory, practices, and future directions. *Contemporary Educational Psychology, 61*, 101860.

Chapter 6

How Can You Make Learning Meaningful, Relevant, and Interesting?

Perry (2011) tells of a student who missed 90 days of school during his freshman year of high school. After attempting to complete his freshman year two more times, he dropped out. Later, he enrolled in and loved an alternative school in which he learned to use complex computer-aided design (CAD) to design a house. He put himself on track to graduate. He said that in his original school, "he was being fed a plate of food he didn't like. So he didn't eat.... [H]e'd always liked to learn but had just never been offered a dish he could stomach," (pp. 64–65). The alternative school changed his perspective. When his school tasks became meaningful and interesting, his learning accelerated.

Meaningful learning is learning that:

- Directly helps accomplish learner's goals in a utilitarian way, like a team manager learning to use a spreadsheet because it will be used to record data for the team.
- Generates interest in most people, like reading stories of scandal, death, and destruction.
- Engages one's anticipation of finding out what happens, like learning who won a military battle.
- Helps one have aesthetic experiences, like understanding a painting in a way that enhances appreciation.
- Helps one gain understanding of one's world, like understanding why a statue was placed in a nearby park.
- Results in products that are directed to a real audience, like writing a persuasive essay for the school newspaper.
- Feels relevant for future pursuits or goals, like learning about biology because you want to become a farmer or physician.

Examples of Meaningfulness

Making learning meaningful often includes having an audience for one's productions. Cole was a 13-year-old leukemia patient in a hospital (Ehret,

DOI: 10.4324/9781003046516-6

2018). He was assigned an English teacher who attempted various approaches to engage him in writing. The teacher attempted to create digital videos with Cole, but that did not work out. Eventually, Cole just wrote, and they were the longest pieces he had ever produced.

> His pediatrician made a bulletin board in the teen room to display patient writing, and, to Cole's delight, he stapled a copy of Cole's story in the center under dye-cut letters that crowned him 'feature writer'.… I could sense his eyes moving toward it every so often while we played videogames together a few feet away.
>
> (p. 64)

Cole's storytelling engaged competence (he felt competent at telling his own story), autonomy (he rejected digital storytelling and chose to write on paper), and belongingness (he connected with others including his Granny, through the bulletin board presentation). The bulletin board gave purpose and meaning to the writing productions.

One teacher noted that students find it meaningful to write about themselves. He assigned them to write at least 80 words about their most memorable moment using descriptions related to their five senses. His students wrote about topics such as seeing their father arrested in the neighborhood check-cashing store, remembering when a cousin was shot and killed, and becoming a father. One child subverted the assignment by writing about not writing the assignment:

> I don't know any memorable moment. Right now I have writer's block, so I don't remember anything to write about. And I'm tired and sleepy. Everyone in the house is sleeping and it is quiet, so I can hear the refrigerator running. Oh, wait! I have something: Since I was bored today, I decided to bite off my fingernails. They smell like skin. They look short, sharp, and crooked. They taste like the medicine I just put on my brother.
>
> (Owens, 2013, p. 175)

Another teacher asked his students to write to him about something beautiful in their lives. They wrote about flowers, butterflies, sunrises and sunsets, pets, and video games. Only one student could not name anything beautiful in her life. The teacher asked her to talk to relatives and people in the neighborhood and ask, "What's something beautiful in your life?" When he next saw her, she reported that her mother said that she the child was beautiful: "My mama told me I was more beautiful than the most beautiful flower" (Markus, 2017, p. 130).

High school teacher Frank McCourt (2005) had an epiphany when he was reading obviously forged excuse notes that were supposedly from parents. He wrote,

Isn't it remarkable, I thought, how they resist any kind of writing assignment in class or at home. They whine and say they're busy and it's hard putting two hundred words together on any subject. But when they forge these excuse notes they're brilliant.... Here was American high school writing at its best—raw, real, urgent, lucid, brief, lying.

(p. 85)

So, he typed up some of the forged parent excuse notes and distributed them to the class as examples. Then, he assigned them to imagine they were parents whose son or daughter needed an excuse for falling behind. Write on, he told them, which they did. His students were mostly religious, so he came up with additional assignments like "An excuse note from Adam to God" or "An excuse note from Eve to God" (p. 87). He described their response:

The heads went down. Pens raced across paper. They could do this with one hand tied behind their backs. With their eyes closed. Secret smiles around the room.... The bell rang, and for the first time in my three and a half years of teaching, I saw high school students so immersed they had to be urged out of the room by friends hungry for lunch.

(p. 87)

McCourt also had his students read *The New York Times* restaurant reviews and talk about their writing structure, language, and details. Then he had students write their own reviews. Students criticized the school cafeteria and raved about local pizzerias and pretzels.

One pizzeria proprietor told students he'd like to meet me and thank me for calling attention to his business and bringing honor to his profession. It was a hell of a thing to think of this teacher with an Irish name encouraging his students to appreciate the finer things in life. Anytime I wanted a pizza, not just a slice but a whole one, the door was wide open and I could have on that pizza anything I wanted, even if he had to send out to a delicatessen for extra toppings he might not have.

(p. 230)

Food is great for grabbing meaningful attention. McCourt once had a student, Kenny, eating marzipan in class. McCourt had never heard of marzipan. Kenny offered to bring in 36 examples so that everyone could try some. Then a different student said he could bring in items from his father's restaurant. A Korean student offered to bring in spicy kimchee. The next day's class became a vocabulary lesson that met in a park using benches to serve the food. They shared with doctors, police, and homeless who were passing by. Everyone needed cold water after the hot and spicy kimchee. And the students learned new things—including vocabulary.

A middle school assigned sixth graders to read *The Immortal Life of Henrietta Lacks*, a *New York Times* bestseller that was certainly not written for sixth graders (Lopez, 2016). It is about a poor Black woman in the 1950s whose cells are easily grown in labs, unlike most people's. The cells have been grown ever since by scientists for medical research on things like the polio vaccine, cancer, and viruses. Progeny of her cells continue to be bought, sold, and used in research. The students broke into groups and analyzed different aspects of the book such as contributions to scientific discoveries, how people made money from Henrietta Lacks' cells without her permission, how civil rights and sexism affected Henrietta Lacks' life, and the ethics of the use of her cells. The topics were meaningful to the students and to contemporary life. The students were able to have their copies of the book signed by the author Rebecca Skloot at an author presentation; author signings would never happen with readings of Shakespeare, Hemingway, or Orwell.

In order to help students see the past as interesting and connected to the present, one history teacher found historical photos of places in town and took contemporary photos from the exact same vantage points (Estes, 2017). A teacher could make similar bids to make school learning meaningful. Find historical photos and assign students to take photos from the same vantage points. Or, assign students to investigate the settings in the photos like who owned old stores or old homes. Have students interview older residents about local events like beauty pageants, sports championships, demolitions, and new construction.

Some interventions to make learning meaningful can backfire. You know the classic winter activity of folding white paper and then cutting it in patterns to make snowflakes? One teacher (Done, 2005) decided to do that activity with flour tortillas, fry the tortillas in butter, and top them with powdered sugar. He got diverted, burned a tortilla, set off the fire alarm, and had to go outside with the rest of the school. Notice the pun on back*fire*!

Instructors can make learning meaningful by connecting new knowledge to valued knowledge. Consider pop music. One can link singers to history and geography. The popular singer Beyoncé is a descendant of Joseph Broussard, who was a leader of the Acadian people. The Acadians were descendants of a French group that settled in eastern Canada (Nova Scotia, New Brunswick, Prince Edward Island, and parts of Quebec). Between 1755 and 1764, because of the French and Indian War, they were expelled by the British from Canada. Many died, and some ended up in today's Louisiana, where they became the Cajuns.

Interview: Make Learning Meaningful

High School Social Studies and Psychology Teacher at a Rural High School. Fourteen Years of Experience

As a social studies teacher I have encountered students who feel that historical events are so far removed from themselves that they have no relevance. I think part of the challenge is that technology affecting our communication & transportation capabilities has changed at an exponential rate in recent decades. It almost feels like time is traveling faster and historical events are farther back than they seem. I assigned an interview project, and several students reported that they really enjoyed the interview with their grandparent or elderly neighbor. Here were people who they saw on a regular basis but never took the time to visit with about their life experiences. I'm teaching a World History course next year, and I'm wondering how I can help students make connections between past civilizations and their lives today. Obviously, there won't be interview candidates, but I think we can still work to help students perceive even ancient history from a new perspective if they understand the ripple effect that civilizations and cultures have upon one another.

Relevance

Making learning relevant is a broad topic that overlaps with meaningfulness and interest and increases motivation. Relevance is often framed as making learning useful for near-term goals like computing shopping costs or for long-term goals like preparing for a future career. Researchers implemented a career relevance intervention for 6th graders in seven schools and continued it through 8th grade. The program strove to show the relevance of the middle grades curriculum by linking school learning to what adults in real jobs and occupations do with information that is being taught in the classroom. The program showed how mathematics, language arts, social studies, and science are used in specific careers (Woolley et al., 2013). The research found that math performance improved; reading performance also improved, but the improvement was not statistically significant. Relevance interventions can motivate students by helping them see that course work is meaningful and useful.

One approach to relevance is utility-value interventions that help students make connections between the material that they are learning and their own lives; utility-value interventions show students that the learned material could be useful now or in the future. Most have the students make the connections between current learning and future value. Here are three key points for utility-value interventions (Hulleman & Harackiewicz, 2021):

1   It is best if the connections are personal and usually made by the learner.
2   The connections need to be specific.
3   The connections need to be directly relevant to the content being learned.

The interventions ask learners to write about connections between the content being learned and their own lives. Two prompts for writing include 1) select a topic from current course content and write about how it connects to your life, and 2) write a letter to another person such as parent, sibling, friend, or fellow student about how course content could be relevant to the other person. For some school topics, students may struggle to make connections between course content and their lives. Teachers should scaffold the connections keeping in mind the background knowledge and experience of the learners. Novices in a field may need more scaffolding than advanced students, and some domains like mathematics may need more scaffolding than domains like nutrition or composition. Evidence suggests that it is best to repeat the writing task more than once but not so often that students get bored.

What outcomes does the utility-value intervention improve? Research shows that it can improve motivation, grades, interest, and course pass rates. Across various studies, the intervention effects were strongest for students who are likely to struggle such as students with poor grades, with lower expectations for success, and from underrepresented groups such as minoritized groups and first-generation college students.

One might expect that it would be more effective if teachers or parents just told students how course content is relevant to their lives, but there is evidence that it is better if students do the thinking and linking. Having students show their own relevance or combining student-generated relevance with teacher-generated relevance worked better than teacher alone (Canning & Harackiewicz, 2015).

The intervention wording for a high school science course included

a   "Pick one of the topics or concepts that we have covered in this unit and briefly summarize the main parts," and
b   "Apply this topic/concept to your life, or to the life of someone you know. How might the information be useful to you, or a friend/relative, in daily life? How does learning about this topic apply to your future plans?"

(Hulleman & Harackiewicz, 2021, p. 111).

A prompt for a biology course gave specific guidance (Hulleman & Harackiewicz, 2021):

1   Select a course concept and formulate a two-part question. Use this question as the title of your essay. A sample question is "What are mutagens and why are they potentially harmful to DNA?"
2   Write a 500 to 600-word essay answering this question and discussing how the information could be useful to you.

Rich Problems

Making learning meaningful does not necessarily mean making learning immediately relevant to everyday life. Meaning and resulting motivation can come from striving to understand. Math educators can use rich problems that motivate students to problem solve but don't have an immediate use. Rich problems are problems that can be solved in multiple ways, and the solutions suggest new questions and new ways of thinking about course content. For example, for a math class, students can figure out the number of squares in a chessboard, meaning *all* the squares, not just the 64 squares that hold chess pieces (Boaler, 2008). Students can use brute force counting, but the problem is rich because additional problems arise from the original problem. For example, after the students solve the number of squares problem, the teacher can challenge students to come up with a way to *compute* the number for an 8 x 8 chessboard. Then the teacher can ask students to generate an equation that allows one to compute the number of squares for boards of different sizes (e.g., 6 x 6 or 12 x 12).

Another example of a rich problem is the magic square (Schoenfeld, 1989). Students are asked to place the numbers 1 through 9 in a 3x3 box so that the sum of the digits in each row, column, and diagonal is the same. The first task is to figure out what is the number that must be the sum for each row, column, and diagonal. (The number is 15 for a 3 x 3 box.) Once they figure that out, students think they are done. But the teacher can ask if certain numbers must appear in certain cells. Could you use the numbers 2 through 10 instead of 1 through 9? Or, what if the square is 4 x 4? What about non-consecutive numbers separated by 5 like 7, 12, 17, 22 …? Let the students come up with more mathematical questions. The students are doing mathematics instead of merely solving a problem whose solution is already known to the teacher. These sorts of problems motivate thinking even though they are not relevant to daily concerns. They can be transformative experiences, our next topic, that change the way that learners see mathematics and numbers.

Transformative Experience

Have you ever learned something that changed how you saw the world? Perhaps you learned about how men tend to talk over women, and now you see that all the time at work. Or, perhaps you learned about negative effects of invasive plant species like kudzu, honey suckle, Bradford pear, and English ivy, and now you look at invasive species with disdain and admire native plants. Or, maybe you learned about what causes the seasons, and now you notice how the height of the sun in the sky changes with the seasons, and you think more carefully about where to place your garden. As we teach, we should be thinking about how our instruction could change the way that learners experience the world. There is an aesthetic dimension to this. That is, new knowledge may not always improve your students' ability to earn money, but it can enhance their quality of life.

In fact, applying what we know can be fun. Helen Czerski (2017), a physicist, described a presentation to business leaders in which she showed a video of two spinning eggs. In the video, a hand stopped both eggs from spinning, but one egg continued to spin slightly. She asked which egg was raw. She said that various members of the audience came up to afterwards to verify that the raw egg continues to move because the liquid contents continue to rotate inside the shell while the hard-boiled egg stops completely. These adults were highly motivated and cried "Yes!" when she verified their hunches. She pointed out that the physics of the spinning egg is used in the Hubble Space Telescope, and she exclaimed,

> The same little physical law we can play with in the kitchen and use, also explains what makes possible some of the most advanced technology of our time! So this is the fun bit of physics, that you learn these patterns and then you can apply them again and again and again. And it's really rewarding when you spot them in new places. This is the fun of physics.

In contrast, Andrea diSessa (2000), a physicist and education researcher, wrote that

> The most disturbing thing I uncovered in a study of bright, motivated, and successful MIT undergraduates years ago was that, although all did well in high school physics and got high marks, almost none felt they really understood the material. Those students' teachers just did not work on intuitive judgments and sense making or connect instruction with ongoing enterprises that the students could own.... Committed learning in such an environment is dead on arrival.
>
> (p. 107)

What can teachers do to help students feel motivated to understand material and connect with their own worlds?

One way to think about these questions is *transformative experience*. Transformative experience refers to situations in which learners newly understand concepts in ways that help them to see and experience their everyday worlds in new ways (Pugh, 2020). Most of the research on transformative experience has been done in science domains. For example, after learning about animal adaptation, a learner might look at their pet dog's teeth with new insight regarding why dogs have teeth that are different from but also similar to human teeth. Transformative experience can be applied to non-science domains. For example, someone who learns about architecture could see that buildings with different styles have different influences that may come from places such as Greece, Germany, and Egypt. Someone who learns about tempo and key in music could hear popular songs with new insight and understanding.

Transformative experience occurs when learners experience the following:

1   motivated use, which refers to application of the learning in free-choice situations. Someone who learns about tempo and key in music does not *have* to hear songs in new ways but can choose to.
2   Expansion of perception, which refers to experiencing the world in new ways as a result of the new knowledge.
3   Experiential value, which refers to valuing the new knowledge because it enriches everyday experience; that is, it has an aesthetic dimension that creates perceptions of artistry in everyday life.

Transformative experience is not the same as transformative learning or life transformation, where someone has an epiphany and totally or partially changes their life, like switching their career, experiencing religious conversion, or deciding to move to a new place (Heddy & Pugh, 2015). Transformative experience is about small insight-producing experiences that change how we perceive the world.

Consider someone in the US who understands science. Their knowledge enriches their experience. When they get up in the morning in late March, they notice that it is darker in the morning because Daylight Savings Time has started (in most states), but the day is longer and the sun is higher in the sky. They understand why. They know where to park their car to catch the morning sun and they know why. They notice that the moon seems to follow the sun across the sky but at a much slower rate, and they know where the moon will rise and set, and they understand why. They understand why in a car crash, holding their arm in front of a small child to prevent their smashing into the dashboard is useless; the child better be belted in. They notice that along a northern river, there are gouges in the upstream side of trees about 4 feet above ground level and know why (in the spring, ice floating in high water bashes into the trees). They under-stand the danger of opening yogurt or fountain pens in airplanes where air pressure is less than at sea level. All of these pieces of knowledge give the person advantages in understanding and also greater aesthetic enjoyment of life.

When Pugh and colleagues (Pugh, Bergstrom, & Spencer, 2017) studied transformative experience in middle school science students who were learning about air pressure, heat transfer, and causes of weather, they found that students fit into high, medium, and low levels of transformative experience. Students in the high group reported transformative experiences like paying more attention to the weather news and being pleased because they understood high and low pressure fronts and what that meant for the weather forecast. One said that when clothes shopping, he thought about the insulation value of different types of clothing and how the insulation might prevent conduction and convection. Another said,

> I think about weather all the time, like I said, I can't get it out of my head. I can't help but think about it. And when I see a lot of things it just affects me 'cause I can't get it out of my head. So it's really affected my life.

(p. 387)

However, there were other students who did not experience motivated use, expansion of perception, or experiential value. A goal for teachers, par-ents, coaches, counselors, and therapists who work with youth should be that learners take what they learn and use it in their daily lives (Pugh & Bergin, 2005).

While research on transformative experience has focused on science education, the same principles apply to learning in any domain. Con-sider the following examples of transformative experience in varied domains:

Literature: Understand literary symbols and use that knowledge to better appreciate films.

- Ripley (Sigorney Weaver) symbolized Christ when falling into a furnace with her arms outstretched at the end of *Alien 3*.
- Ice symbolized frozen hearts in the film *Frozen*.

Science: Understand science principles and recognize how they apply in everyday life.

- How a double walled water bottle keeps liquids warm or cold.
- Why a piece of marble in a warm room feels cool even though it is the same temperature as everything else in the room.

Architecture: Distinguish architectural styles and apply that knowledge in cities and neighborhoods.

- Recognize Queen Anne home characteristics such as asymmetrical structure, wraparound porch, tower or turret, wood shingles that resemble fish scales. (See Figure 6.1)
- Recognize Gothic church characteristics such as pointed (ogival) arches, ribbed vaults, and stained glass. Notre Dame in Paris is an example.

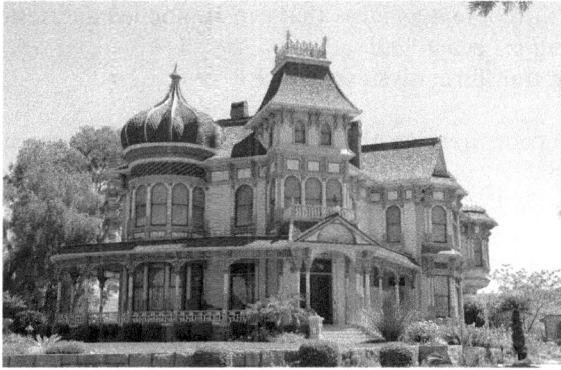

Figure 6.1

Foreign language: Learn words and phrases in a foreign language.

- Recognize words and phrases in film.
- Learn to use the subjunctive in Spanish or French and then recognize that English has a subjunctive voice.

Physics: Understand key principles of physics.

- Realize that if someone drops an object from a high building or bridge, the object will not continue to fall faster and faster; friction with the air (drag) and other factors such as weight and surface area can reduce speed.
- Understand that heat rises, which helps you know where you should place fuel to build up a fire.

Music: Distinguish musical structures.

- Recognize guitar riffs and recognize the same riffs in varied types of music.
- Understand how major and minor keys, syncopation, and beat affect mood and emotion; recognize them in songs.

Social Studies/History: Recognize how historical events are repeated.

- The fall of Afghanistan in 2021 is like the fall of Vietnam in 1975.
- Hitler's attempt to invade Russia in 1941 was like Napoleon's attempt to invade Russia in 1812. Both attempts failed.

Teaching for Transformative Experiences in Science (TTES, Pugh, Bergstrom, Heddy, et al., 2017) is a model that suggests three teaching behaviors:

1 framing the content as ideas that can be applied and tested,
2 scaffolding re-seeing, and
3 modeling transformative experience.

The first behavior, framing the content, can include metaphors or pithy statements that awaken anticipation about seeing and experiencing the world differently. For example, Girod and Wong (2002) used the metaphor "Every rock is a story waiting to be read" as a way of teaching geology and encouraging students to look at rocks in a new way. This resulted, for example, in Brieana's statement, "I wasn't all that interested in rocks before, but now I am. I used to pick them up at the beach and throw them in the water. Now, I couldn't throw all those stories away" (p. 212). A teacher referred to "weather as a recipe" in order to encourage students to think about the "ingredients" that result in different weather patterns (Pugh et al., 2017). A teacher referred to plants and animals as stories that are waiting to be read in order to encourage students to think about adaptation to environments, such as different bird beaks and different mammal camouflage patterns (Pugh et al., 2010).

The second behavior, scaffolding re-seeing, emphasizes helping students see an entity in a new way. Even if students develop anticipation about seeing the world in a new way, they may struggle to do so and need support. Re-seeing can include assignments like the teacher who asked students to "read" animals "by discussing their unique characteristics and the purpose of these characteristics" (Pugh et al., 2010, p. 290). In response, a student commented on the large eyes of owls. Students could also comment on things like what type of teeth do animals like wolves and bears have? Why? Could they learn to eat grain and grass? Is that similar to cats? How do the teeth compare to humans or robins? Another teacher assigned students to share dramatic weather experiences like a very windy day and then make a presentation on how a simple weather experience could be re-seen by thinking about air pressure and weather fronts (Pugh, Bergstrom, & Spencer, 2017).

The third behavior, modeling transformative experience, involves the teacher describing personal experience with motivated use, expansion of perception, and experiential value. For example, a teacher described his experience with opening a yogurt cup—and the ensuing spurt of yogurt—at an altitude higher than where the yogurt was packaged (Pugh et al., 2017). A teacher could describe how knowledge of Shakespeare might influence responses to movies like *10 Things I Hate About You, She's the Man*, or *The Lion King*. A musician could comment on how the "Bo Diddley beat" influenced their perceptions of rock and roll songs like Springsteen's *She's the One* and many others (Pappas, 2019). A film fan could comment on how African style and art influenced their perceptions of Beyonce's *Lemonade* (Okoroafor, 2016) and the film *Black Panther* (Chutel & Kazeem, 2018). It is important that the teacher explain his or her experience, not preach to the students about what their experience ought to be. This should be a modeling activity, not a didactic lesson. And the modeling should include explication of the aesthetic richness that comes from understanding what influenced the events that were experienced.

An adult *New York Times* reporter reflected on a mathematics experience that changed how she saw mathematics and the world:

> When I was ten years old I had what I can only describe as a mystical experience. It came during a math class. We were learning about circles, and to his eternal credit our teacher, Mr. Marshall, let us discover for ourselves the secret image of this unique shape: the number known as pi. Almost everything you want to say about circles can be said in terms of pi, and it seemed to me in my childhood innocence that a great treasure of the universe had just been revealed. Everywhere I looked I saw circles, and at the heart of every one of them was this mysterious number. It was in the shape of the sun and the moon and the earth; in mushrooms, sunflowers, oranges, and pearls; in wheels, clock faces, crockery, and telephone dials. All of these things were united by pi, yet it transcended them all. I was enchanted. It was as if someone had lifted a veil and shown me a glimpse of a marvelous realm beyond the one I experienced with my senses. From that day on I knew I wanted to know more about the mathematical secrets hidden in the world around me.
>
> (as cited in Boaler, 2008, pp. 18–19)

Interview: Transformative Experience

High School Social Studies and Psychology Teacher at a Rural High School. Fourteen Years of Experience

As a Psychology teacher, it is my goal to help students understand that our mental health and functioning impacts every aspect of our life. I often refer to this as a "psychology switch" that, once we flip on, they won't be able to turn back off; they will begin seeing psychological concepts we learn about in the classroom everywhere around them! I loved reading the article on transformative experiences because I think this ability to "see & experience their everyday worlds in new ways" is exactly what I've been referring to as a "psychology switch."

For example, we begin with a Memory Unit in my Psychology of the Brain & AP Psychology classes. In this unit, we learn various models for how our brains encode, store, & retrieve information as well as strategies and processes that allow us to utilize our memories more effectively. I ask the students why we begin the semester with this unit even though it's buried further within our textbook. They usually answer, "Because we're going to have a lot of stuff to remember in this class!" We laugh a bit & then expound on that answer. I ask them what sort of things they think they're going to have to remember for the course & whether they will be the same types of things they have to remember for other classes. We expound beyond traditional classroom experiences as well & discuss the role of memory in sports, the arts, relationships, etc. I will often have students share examples throughout the unit of how learning about our memory systems has impacted them. Some have shared mnemonic strategies they utilized to learn material in science they were struggling with. Others have put spaced practice into application for their academic studies because they see how powerful it is in sports or music practice schedules. One of the most powerful (& heart-wrenching) examples was when a student shared how their grandparent's struggle with dementia revealed to them that even our most significant relationships are essentially a compilation of memories of experiences we have compiled over time & that the erosion of that memory trace also erodes the relationship. The fact that students are sharing these experiences voluntarily illustrates that (1) they are motivated to use the information we are learning, (2) their perception of life experiences is changing because of what they've learned, and (3) their new perspective is valuable because it helps them navigate their world more richly.

In order to help students have these transformative experiences throughout the year, I want to begin thinking of each unit in terms of the model for Teaching for Transformative Experiences in Science. I can model my own experience of transitioning from a fixed to a growth mindset by sharing examples of how I used to cry in class when I didn't understand a problem because I was embarrassed that I would never be able to solve it. Later I learned to calm myself by visualizing myself on the other side of the challenge having successfully coped with it; I understood it was too difficult for me at that moment, but I had the strategies and resources to tackle it.

Interest

Interest is often separated into individual interest and situational interest. Individual interest refers long-standing interest that a person has developed over time, like an interest in pop singers of the 1990s. Situational interest refers to interest that arises from a particular situation, like a chemistry teacher lighting balloons on fire. One way to think about the two types of interest is that factors that are largely under teacher control (like using humor) are situation factors, whereas factors that are difficult to change (like background knowledge) or nearly impossible to change (like students' cultural background) are individual factors (Bergin, 1999).

In the short term, teachers have little influence on individual interests, but they can take advantage of them to motivate. This is especially true if there are individual interests that most or many students have in common. Such interests can be regional or specific to racial-ethnic status. For example, in rural areas, students might be interested in agriculture, farm vehicles, horses, crop growing, and related topics; some topics may be especially, but not uniquely, true of males or females. Some sports are more popular in certain geographical areas, like basketball, football, lacrosse, fishing, etc. A teacher should be attuned to interests that generally exist in a community.

A teacher should also be aware of individual interests that are unique to individuals. Just because video games or pop music are popular does not mean that every individual holds that interest. Individuals can be quite idiosyncratic, like the boy who dances ballet or the girl who boxes. It takes attention and persistence to discover individual interests. Some youth are anxious to share their interests with everyone, but others are more private and less likely to share. Knowing students' individual interests can be relevant to fostering belongingness by showing awareness of their interests. Knowing can also influence instruction because the astute teacher will make references to students' interests and draw their attention. For example, a physics teacher might know that certain students are interested in video games or Wii-style fitness games and discuss how the games must use algorithms to compute the trajectory of vehicles, tennis balls, and thrown objects like knives. An English teacher might know that certain students love the current blockbuster series (like Harry Potter or the Twilight series) and invite them to compare the vocabulary and prose style of the current bestseller with a classic literary work that they are studying. The more that teachers know about their students' individual interests, the more they can customize their curriculum and foster motivation.

Situational interests tend to be relatively global in the sense that they involve topics that would grab most people's interest. Wade and colleagues (1993) claimed that "topics related to injury, sex, and scandal are clearly of high interest to readers almost without exception. In other words, such topics do appear to have absolute, or inherent, interest across readers, evoking a kind of emotional interest" (p. 106). Schank (1979) wrote that death, unexpected events, and danger are interesting in most cases. Teachers can choose tasks and experiences that are likely to generate situational interest (Bergin, 1999). Teachers (and zoos) often find that topics such as dinosaurs, marine mammals (e.g., whales, seals, sea otters), and pandas attract widespread interest. Teachers can use hands-on activities, novelty, games, puzzles, fantasy, humor, and stories to attract attention.

Educators who increase their use of interesting tasks should think carefully because attempts to attract interest can distract from learning and thus *reduce* learning. For example, hands-on activities can lead to students mainly playing with materials and having fun rather than engaging the learning goals of the activity. One researcher (Zahorik, 1996) commented that

> Of the interesting activities that were described, at least one-third were hands-on activities that seemed gratuitous in whole or in part. They probably generated much interest, but whether they led to the acquisition of important learning is unclear. Hands-on activities appeared to be only loosely related to content objectives.... The hands-on activities of the 1950s units were to sing Elvis songs, impersonate Elvis, write essays speculating on whether Elvis was still alive, and critique Elvis movies.
>
> (p. 556)

A classroom study found that identifying the contents of owl pellets resulted in much time spent "separating, artistically arranging, and gluing bones" (Blumenfeld & Meece, 1988, p. 244) rather than on understanding the point of the lesson, which was animal adaptation. The same study observed another class that focused on how to do and understand experiments. The task was to figure out what colors attracted mealy worms. The students spent much time "comparing how fast their worms moved, how much they wiggled, or exchanging worms for ones that were fatter, bigger, or quicker" (p. 244) rather than on understanding how to run an experiment and analyze data. Educators should carefully consider the degree to which an interesting lesson will foster learning versus messing around.

There is evidence that drawing attention to irrelevant but interesting features of instruction can detract from learning. This has been demonstrated by research on seductive details, which are elements of instruction that present interesting but unimportant information (Garner et al., 1989). The authors of a meta-analysis of seductive details (Sundararajan & Adesope, 2020) used the example of a lesson about the causes of volcanoes. The teacher described the historic 1815 eruption of Mount Tabora in Indonesia to grab attention, but the description told nothing about the causes of volcanoes, which was the point of the lesson. Thus, the description of ash that darkened the sun and reduced light for plants, causing starvation and disease, was disturbing and interesting but not instructionally useful. The negative effects seem to occur because seductive details distract attention from the instructional purpose, disrupt the students' ability to create a coherent mental representation, and activate irrelevant prior knowledge. Teachers should clearly frame their lessons in interesting ways, but they need to guide the students to see how the interesting details support, rather than detract from, key instructional points.

Case 6.1

Alice, a child with high functioning autism, was observed at ages 8, 11, and 13. She developed interests in skeletons, animals, fossils, and mechanical things (Sjödin, 2015). She was very precise, and if a teacher or classmate made a statement that was not precisely correct, Alice would correct them. A teacher objected, saying, "We've been trying to explain to her that it is not acceptable. She has to understand that she cannot do things like that" (p. 90). A teacher objected to Alice's intense interests because they took up too much time, distracted her from the curriculum, and disrupted school routine: "it is more important that she completes the same five pages of math as everyone else" (p. 91). Teachers reported that Alice resisted activities that she perceived as meaningless: "If she does not understand why she should do something, she does not even try" (p. 91). A teacher said that "It is good for these children to be a little bored. They benefit from it" (p. 91). What do you think about Alice and teachers' attitudes toward her in light of motivation concepts of meaningfulness, autonomy, achievement goals, and interest? How does her autism factor into your thoughts?

Mystery and Suspense

Robert Cialdini, researcher and author of the best seller *Influence: The Psychology of Persuasion*, wrote that a key to keeping student attention is to introduce mysteries and puzzles into instruction. He wrote, "Mystery stories do not need personal relevance—they bring their own. Mystery stories bring their own relevance in the form of a need for closure that most everyone shares to some degree" (Cialdini, 2005, p. 24). He gave two major examples. First, what are the Rings of Saturn made of? Cambridge University scientists claimed they were made of gas; a group at MIT said dust particles; a group at Cal Tech claimed ice crystals. An effective lesson would pose questions so that students wonder what are they really made of and anxiously anticipate the answer (ice-covered dust, but mostly dust).

Second, why did the tobacco industry propose banning tobacco ads from television and radio even as their sales were dropping? This seems counterintuitive, and a lesson could keep students wondering why until late in the lesson. (US law required that equal advertising space had to be granted to all sides of important and controversial topics; this applied to tobacco use, but only on radio and television. Anti-tobacco ads were broadcast for no cost by groups like the American Cancer Society so that they could respond to the tobacco industry's paid advertising. Therefore, the tobacco industry thought it best to appear benevolent by agreeing to ban advertising on radio and television.)

Effective teachers can come up with mysteries in their own fields. Some suggestions include the following:

- Martin Luther King, Jr. had a different name at birth. What was it and why did it change?
- What makes bread dough rise?
- When you put ice in a glass of water, how does the water get through the glass to create water drips on the outside?
- If you put an apple in a cooler with dry ice, why does the apple get carbonated?
- If you go up a hill at 20 mph and the same distance down the hill at 60 mph, what is your average speed? (as mentioned earlier, 30 mph) Why is it not 40 mph?
- Daniel Ortega was a leader in the Nicaraguan revolution against dictator Anastasio Somoza in 1979 and by 1985 was the president of Nicaragua. To what degree did Ortega retain his revolutionary ideals? What happened to Somoza?
- In 1993, indigenous peoples in the Ecuadorian Amazon sued Texaco/Chevron for polluting their lands. Did they get money for cleanup?

Cialdini asserts that the instructor needs to avoid the typical approach of describing what happens or posing a question and answering it. The instructor needs to get the students to participate in creating an explanation of the phenomenon. The instructor provides information and clues, but the students generate the explanation.

Teachers can elicit suspense by the way that they present information. Students in history class are not likely to know if John J. Pershing caught Pancho Villa, or who won the battle at Vicksburg, or did Marie Antoinette survive the French Revolution. You could tell those stories as suspenseful narratives that withhold the outcomes until the end instead of dry bullet-pointed presentations. Science demonstrations can suspensefully *show* what happens, for example, when cotton in an inverted cup is thrust into water and comes out dry, and then explain why, instead of *telling* what happens and then demonstrating it with no suspense. The demonstration could be live or via video, like the video of a feather and bowling ball being dropped at the same time in a vacuum (they hit the ground at the same time; search YouTube for videos on feather bowling ball drop) or the video of a bullet being dropped and another fired at the same time from the same height (which hits the ground first? They hit at the same time. Why? Search YouTube for Mythbusters bullet drop). The suspense effect is enhanced when you ask students to make a prediction; then they are committed to an outcome and want to see if it happens. There can be elements of suspense in many domains.

Art: What happens when you mix different colors of paint (what color will emerge)? What happens when you mix colored light (is it the same as mixing paint)?

Social and behavioral science: Is the teen birth rate increasing? Which country has the highest math test scores and how have they changed over 50 years? Do financial incentives improve performance?

Math: If you folded a piece of paper 42 times, how thick would it be? Is it true that every even whole number greater than 2 is the sum of two prime numbers (the Goldbach conjecture)?

In the classroom, most suspense will be of the observational type in which the instructor tells a story (who will win the historical battle?) or demonstrates an effect (what will happen when the concoction is heated?). Suspense of the participatory type can be invoked through competition, the next chapter.

Research and Theory into Practice

Many topics in this book are relevant to creating relevance, interest, and meaningfulness. Table 6.1 presents some approaches that you can use.

Table 6.1. Research-based methods for promoting interest, relevance, and meaningfulness

Method	Explanation
Build competence and confidence	Students feel more interest and motivation when they feel competent. This applies to domains such as academics, social interaction, selecting careers, diet control, exercise, and so forth. Self-efficacy leads to increased motivation, which leads to effort and improved skills, which leads to improved performance.
Build on background knowledge	People tend to be interested in things that they know about, and the more they learn, the more interested they become. Find out what your learners and clients know about and are interested in. Activate that knowledge.

Method	Explanation
Use active learning in which learners DO something	Learners *like* hands-on activities, role playing, problem-solving activities, and building things. Active learning needs to also be minds-on, focusing student thinking on the topic to be learned. Classroom response systems like clickers can be helpful in classroom settings.
Use rewards, but sparingly	Learners' motivation may be increased by rewards when they have no prior interest. Sometimes, as students engage in a task for a reward, they develop competence and increased motivation. The next chapter describes a teen who was not interested in running, was paid to participate in cross-country, and ended up liking running. Rewards can undermine *intrinsic* motivation if learners are already interested in a topic.
Use praise, but carefully	Praise can foster motivation if it fosters perceptions of competence and gives feedback about how to improve. It can undermine motivation if it seems controlling and undermines autonomy.
Present learners with a discrepancy	Learners tend to become interested when told something that they think is true is actually false. They are motivated to resolve the discrepancy. This is relevant to instruction, therapy, and coaching. For example, most people think the cause of the seasons is the distance from the sun, but the earth is usually closest to the sun in January, the northern hemisphere's winter. Athletes may think that more and more training is useful, but it can lead to over-training and injury.
Tell a good story	Learners find narratives and stories more interesting and motivating than analytic, expository text. Use stories in instruction, therapy, and coaching. Mystery stories are especially engaging. Avoid stories that are irrelevant or distracting.
Use suspense	Teachers can read a book to the class, and then quit at a cliffhanger event so the students have to read it themselves to find out what happens. Coaches can tell about companies or teams that implemented changes and then suspensefully work up to what happened.
Explain the value or relevance of the activity	Learners and clients want to know how they might benefit from a task or exercise. The instructor or interventionist should explain relevance.
Have learners generate reasons or goals for their activity	Research shows that it can be effective for motivation and learning to have the learners figure out the relevance.

Summary

- Meaningful learning has utility, generates interest, creates anticipation, fosters aesthetic experience, fosters understanding, creates products for an audience, and is relevant to personal goals.
- Learning relevant to personal goals increases motivation.
- Utility-value interventions show relevance by helping students see that the learned material could be useful now or in the future. Relevance can be shown by an instructor or can be generated by learners.
- Rich problems are motivating and foster deep learning but don't necessarily have an immediate use.
- Transformative experience refers to situations in which learners newly understand concepts in ways that help them to see and experience their everyday worlds in new ways. They occur when learners experience

  a   Motivated use, which refers to using the learning when you don't have to.

  b   Expansion of perception, which refers to experiencing the world in new ways as a result of the new knowledge.

  c   Experiential value, which refers to valuing the new knowledge because it enriches everyday experience.

- Individual interest refers long-standing interest that a person has developed over time. Instructors have little short-term influence on individual interest.
- Situational interest refers to interest that arises from a particular situation and can be introduced by instructors.
- Fostering interest increases learning and motivation, but some interesting tasks can distract and thus *reduce* learning.
- Suspense and mystery can foster motivation and learning.

Suggestions for Further Reading

Bergin, D. A. (1999). Influences on classroom interest. *Educational Psychologist, 34*(2), 87–98.

Middleton, M., & Perks, K. (2014). *Motivation to Learn*. Corwin.

Pugh, K. J. (2020). *Transformative Science Education: Change How your Students Experience the World*. Teachers College Press.

Willingham, D. T. (2009). *Why Don't Students Like School?* Jossey-Bass.

Chapter 7

How Does Competition Affect Motivation?

Competition refers to a situation in which two or more individuals or groups vie for a goal that only one can achieve. People compete all the time for jobs, mates, housing, fame, and credit. For example, scientists compete to be first with inventions and to get credit for their inventions; scientists compete to be awarded prizes like the Nobel Prize (about $1 million), the Breakthrough Prize in Life Sciences ($3 million), and the Kavli Prize ($1 million). People in sales compete to sell more. I have talked with teachers who competed for better student test scores. High school students compete for test scores and to be valedictorian. I once talked with a high school student who graduated a year early because she knew she would be valedictorian of the earlier cohort but not the later. Politicians compete to be elected. Athletes compete to win. Musicians compete to be first chair. Children filling out worksheets compete to be the first to finish. Teachers and schools sometimes create competition among students because they believe that competition will create greater motivation. However, competition needs to be considered carefully because it can foster motivation or undermine motivation.

US schools seem to be particularly competitive. The 2018 Programme for International Student Assessment asked students whether they cooperated or competed and whether they valued cooperation and competition. The US ranked as one of the countries where students reported high level of competition relative to cooperation (Programme for International Student Assessment, 2020). Is that good or bad? It depends. In the following sections, I will discuss the good, the bad, and the mixed about competition.

The Bad of Competition

Kohn (1992) wrote an entire book criticizing competition. He pointed out that people, especially Americans, often believe the following myths:

- Competition is unavoidable because it is part of human nature.
- Competition motivates humans to do their best.
- Competition is the best way to have a good time.

DOI: 10.4324/9781003046516-7

- Competition builds character and is good for self-confidence.

Kohn wrote that competition is not part of human nature, does not improve performance, is not a good way to have a good time, and does not build character; in fact, it might undermine character. Kohn did not see competition as having redeemable qualities: "The more closely I have examined the topic, the more firmly I have become convinced that competition is an inherently undesirable arrangement, that the phrase *healthy competition* is actually a contradiction in terms."

Some of the negative effects of competition that Kohn describes include the following:

- A reduction in intrinsic motivation as participants focus on winning rather than on doing the activity.
- Overall reduction in academic achievement and other measures of performance.
- A reduction in the quality of performance as participants cut corners and even cheat to win.
- A belief that some people are winners and some are losers.
- Pressure to try to best others instead of enjoying their company or cooperating with them.
- A belief that success means beating others.
- More resources for the "winners" but reduced resources for the "losers."
- Deriving satisfaction from besting other people.
- Pure pleasure of play is replaced by desire to achieve victory through beating everyone else.
- Reduction in youth who play sports because most don't win and therefore lose.
- The "spectacle of frantic, frothing parents humiliating their children in their quest for vicarious triumph."
- An increase in aggression, teasing, and taunts.
- Resentment toward the winners and disparagement of the losers.
- An increase in anxiety due to apprehension about losing or about actually losing.
- A tendency toward conformity because it is difficult to win if you are overly creative, innovative, or risk-taking.

Over the years, there have been various reviews of the effects of competition, and they typically show that competition has negative or neutral effects; on average, competition does not improve performance. A 1980 review (Gorney & Long, 1980) compared cultures to see if competitive cultures were more productive; they were not. A 1981 meta-analysis (Johnson et al., 1981) of 122 studies found that "cooperation is considerably more effective than interpersonal competition and individualistic efforts" (p. 47). This finding was consistent across subject areas (language arts, reading, math, science, social studies, psychology, physical education). A study of psychologists (Helmreich et al., 1980) found that those who were more competitive had fewer citations (how often a psychologist is cited by other psychologists is a measure of success or prominence). Helmreich and colleagues sought more data on this topic. Kohn cites seven of their studies, and all found a negative relationship between competition and performance, participants in the studies were PhD scientists, academic psychologists, 5th and 6th graders, males in business, college students, airline pilots, and airline reservation agents. A more recent meta-analysis (Murayama & Elliot, 2012) of different types of competition found no overall relation between competition and performance.

Consider a 4th-grade teacher who wants to foster reading. She gives the students a form on which they list each book they read. She says that whoever reads 50 books first will get a gift certificate at the local toy store. The first night, Sally's father encourages her to read *Charlotte's Web*, a relatively lengthy chapter book. When she gets to school the next day, she has read half of a book while other, more strategic, students have read ten baby books such as board books with one word per page, like Cow, Horse, and Pig. Meanwhile, the non-readers who are the target of the contest have read zero books. They have spent four to five years learning that they don't like to read, they don't read well, and they look dumb when reading compared to their high-achieving classmates. Do you think that they will now go home and say to themselves, "I am so motivated to compete for the prize"? An additional effect of the competition is that some students will cheat by listing books that they have not read.

You may object that the contest can be improved. For example, the teacher could give smaller prizes for every five books and a big prize to everyone who reads 50 books. But that is much more expensive for the teacher, who is probably paying out of pocket, and it is no longer a competition. Or the teacher could require verification of reading each book to prevent cheating, but that would require a lot of paperwork. In sum, this sort of competition is not motivating for good readers or poor readers because the good readers would read anyway—they are already motivated—and the poor readers check out of the competition.

Competition has been criticized as undermining motivation and performance because there are invariably more losers than winners, and losing tends to make people want to quit. While some people redouble their efforts after a loss, many view a series of losses as evidence that they lack the ability to compete in a domain, so they drop out of the activity.

Many youth are pressured into competing. Schools or parents may require students to participate in competitions such as science fairs, sports, band, and academics (quiz bowl, MathCounts, etc.). For example, a survey of junior high science fair participants found that 35% were required to participate and 70% received extra credit to participate (Abernathy & Vineyard, 2001). A problem with compulsory competition is that compulsion tends to undermine motivation for an activity. Recall from research on autonomy that people participate in activities with a higher quality of motivation when they feel autonomous in their participation, even if they are not intrinsically motivated (Ryan & Deci, 2000). When they are compelled to participate, the quality of their participation is lower than if they chose to compete.

The Good of Competition

Competitions can generate interest and motivation. The prominent mathematician, Herbert Robbins, said that he was not personally interested in mathematics as a college student. He was talked into participating in the Putnam competition, which is a mathematics competition for university students that is so difficult that the median score is often zero. Afterwards, he had a change of heart regarding mathematics and said, "I would never have studied more than a year of mathematics, much less have become ... a mathematician, were it not for the Putnam competition" (Alexanderson et al., 1985, p. xii). Robbins' story is not unique. There are many accounts of youth who developed or intensified their interests as a result of competition (e.g., Dutton, 2011; Olson, 2004). When individuals participate in competition, their interest may grow because they develop competence and meet people who have similar interests.

For example, there are various international Olympiads such as math, physics, and chemistry. A book (Olson, 2004) about the math Olympiad highlighted Melanie Wood, who was an excellent student in all areas. She had never heard of MathCounts, a US competition for students in grades 6–8. Nevertheless, the team coach at her school had heard that she was in an advanced math class and invited her to participate in a competition. She finished first. The team then went to the Indiana State competition, and she finished first. At the national competition, she finished 40 out of 228 competitors. The next year, she finished tenth. In high school, she was on the US Olympiad team that finished third, and the next year that finished ninth. Today, she holds professorships in mathematics at Harvard and UC Berkeley. Would she have pursued mathematics as a profession without the MathCounts competition? There is no way to know, but the competition clearly highlighted to her and others her remarkable talents in mathematics.

Students who prepare for MathCounts and other competitions pore over mathematics books and problems in order to hone their skills (Olson, 2004). It is hard to believe that most would put in that level of effort without competition. One 8th grader "bought several books of Olympiad-level problems and began working his way through them. Sometimes he would struggle over a single problem for hours, but he told himself that it was good training" (p. 85). He took a college math course and studied his father's old college textbooks. This is not a unique pattern. Many if not most of the contestants had similar strategies and motivation for improvement. At the same time, it is important to point out that students could work and work to make the Olympiad team that would go to the international competition, but only six make the team per country. "All those who don't make the team, a group that includes some of the best high school mathematicians in the country, may end up feeling like losers" (p. 87). To my knowledge, no one has written a book about them, so we don't know if they redouble their efforts for the next year or quit.

People who have studied the Olympiads over the years (Campbell & Walberg, 2010) found that most Olympians and their parents believe that they would not have accomplished as much as they did without participation in the Olympiads. Nearly all also believed that the competition did not hinder their development. The authors stated,

> To do well the student must accumulate extensive subject matter knowledge to the point where he or she is able to understand the current research literature and analyze problems confronting scientists, engineers, and mathematicians in that domain. This acquisition of knowledge takes months or even years to assemble. This acquisition of knowledge causes these students to leapfrog over their high-school peers.
>
> (p. 10)

The authors pointed out that the non-winners also acquire extensive knowledge and skills that are relevant to their future careers.

A student who won second place in the ISEF science fair competition had not thought about college because his parents could not afford it (Dutton, 2011). After his science fair success, he won a full ride scholarship to college, went to medical school, and became an obstetrician. Without the science fair, he probably would not have attended college at all. Students who participate in competitions are motivated to learn the content of their field, learn to write better, learn public speaking, learn how to display data in charts and graphs, and learn to construct instruments and apparatus. One science fair enthusiast raised funds for a fair after the regional fair was cancelled, was interviewed by the FBI for photographing a chemical plant (breach of homeland security), built a lab in a trailer on the family lot, earned a patent, won a college scholarship, and was featured on bags of spicy Doritos (Dutton, 2011). She developed extensive skills that she would not have developed otherwise.

People are often motivated to compete spontaneously and informally. Students ask each other what they got on exams; they bet milkshakes about who will get the highest score. When asked what they would do if the school did not compute their GPA or class rank, one student said, "We'd do it ourselves I'm sure" (Bergin & Cooks, 2000, p. 456). Furthermore, students often report enjoying competition. If no one enjoyed competition, there would not be so many formal competitions.

Many organizations host academic STEM competitions. These include Envirothon; Math League; Intel International Science and Engineering Fair; Siemens Competition in Math, Science and Technology; FIRST Robotics Competition; International Science and Mathematical Olympiads; and the Mandelbrot Competition, to name a few. Wankat (2005, 2007) listed 53 engineering-oriented competitions for K-12 students and 44 engineering and technology competitions for undergraduate students. In addition to STEM competitions, there are competitions for fishing, entrepreneurship, speech and debate, music performance, essay writing, and hundreds more. The Scripps National Spelling Bee is even televised.

Institutions like the Scripps media company, US Department of Defense, universities, National Science Foundation, and many others help plan and host competitions because they believe that competitions foster motivation. They believe that preparing for and participating in these competitions fosters interest that leads students to learn (Abernathy & Vineyard, 2001; Bishop & Walters, 2007). When people engage in competitions, they push achievements upward. Youth who hate homework prepare for competition doing the equivalent of many hours of homework—studying, practicing, and quizzing in order to prepare. Ericsson, the expert on expertise, pointed out that procedures for deliberate practice are often best developed in domains that have competitions because the competitions push people to develop better forms of practice. Fields that have competitions have pushed achievements forward. Anglers have benefitted from techniques honed in competitions. Runners have benefitted from shoes that were developed for competitions. In fact, new technologies, strategies, and techniques often emerge from competitions.

Why do people compete? Many competitors freely choose to participate based upon their interest, perceptions of competence, value of the activity (e.g., winning will enhance one's perceptions of competence and might result in a scholarship), social goals (friends are also doing it), and goals to be superior compared to others. Recall that self-determination theory emphasizes the importance of people having the freedom to choose an activity even if the activity is not intrinsically motivated. Individual interest is more likely to develop if competitors freely choose to compete and are not coerced; nevertheless, some may develop interest after being coerced into competition, as Herbert Robbins the mathematician did. In fact, we had a friend who told his couch-potato video-game-playing son that he would pay the son $500 if he joined the cross-country team and finished the season. The son turned out to be pretty good at cross country, earned $500, and stayed on the team the next year without payment. Some reluctant participants in competitions find that their interest is piqued, their social group is expanded, and they begin the process of interest development.

Stage Challenge was a performing arts competition for secondary school youth in New Zealand. A study at a girl's school (Trayes et al., 2012) found that girls who chose to participate reported positive feelings about the Stage Challenge process. They tended not to focus on the competition itself, but on the following: mostly positive emotion with some boredom and frustration; flow, which refers to experience in which you are completely immersed in an activity and lose track of time and of the self; being their authentic selves; performing live; social interaction that included existing and new friends; and accomplishing goals. Notice how these themes fit with topics that have been discussed in this book. For example, autonomy involves being able to engage in behavior that conforms to one's authentic self. Belongingness is a fundamental need for humans and can be manifest in social interaction. Goals are fundamental for motivation. The girls reported that the practices were the worst aspect of the overall experience, which fits with the claim that deliberate practice may not be enjoyable. This is an example of youth choosing a competitive experience and reporting liking it and benefiting from it.

As mentioned earlier, competition can generate suspense because the outcome of the competition is unknown. The element of suspense can make competition enjoyable and motivating (Moulard et al., 2019), especially if the competition is close.

"It Depends" Aspects of Competition

The outcomes of competition depend on your goals. A meta-analysis of dozens of quantitative studies (Murayama & Elliot, 2012) found that overall, competition was not related to performance because the influence of competition depends on achievement goals. The study pointed out that when people are faced with competition, they tend to adopt a performance approach or performance avoidance goal. Recall that the concept of achievement goals was brought up in Chapter 2. One of the achievement goals is a performance approach goal, which is a goal to look better than other people and demonstrate one's ability. This is essentially a competitive goal and an approach goal. Approach goals motivate going after something while avoidance goals motivate avoiding something. Approach goals tend to be associated with positive outcomes and avoidance goals tend to be associated with negative outcomes. The meta-analysis showed that performance depends on whether learners adopt performance approach versus performance avoidance goals. If they adopt performance approach goals, they tend to have high performance compared to those who adopt performance avoidance goals. Chapter 2 pointed out that it is better for students to have performance approach goals than avoidance goals. This finding helps explain why.

The outcomes of competition depend on whether you chose to compete. Recall from the section on autonomy that motivation and performance are improved when people have choice. Youth motivation is usually better if a youth chooses to join the football team, MathCounts team, or dance squad compared to if they are forced to join. In self-chosen activities, if there are aversive events like practicing on hot summer days, losing, or being criticized, the youth thinks "Well, I chose to do this." That contrasts with being forced into a situation where the youth experiences aversive events.

Research has shown that competition increases interest and motivation for winners and for individuals who are strongly achievement-oriented (Epstein & Harackiewicz, 1992; Reeve & Deci, 1996; Song et al., 2013; Tauer & Harackiewicz, 1999; Vansteenkiste & Deci, 2003). While losing sometimes undermines interest and motivation, one study found that providing positive feedback to losers (e.g., even though you lost, you did better than 70% of previous participants) tended to maintain intrinsic motivation in a competitive setting (Vansteenkiste & Deci, 2003).

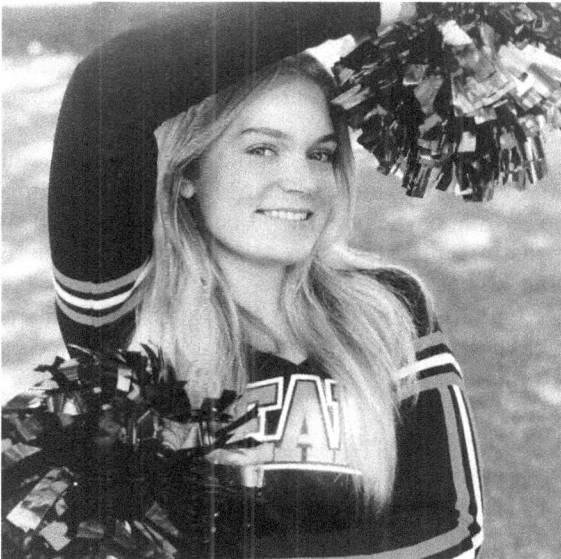

Many settings such as high school basketball teams, high school cheer leading squads, travel soccer teams, theater productions, and others have selective teams; that is, you must compete in a tryout or exam to participate. The emotional effects of the competition depend on whether you are selected or rejected. For example, a study of high school girls who tried out for dance and cheerleading teams found that the not-chosen girls reported feeling negative emotions about themselves and about school compared to the chosen (Barnett, 2007). Teachers reported lower attendance and classroom performance for the not-chosen. Interviews with a subset of 18 chosen and 19 not-chosen found stark differences (Barnett, 2006). Chosen girls were *ecstatic, elated, excited, high*, and *awesome* and said they wanted to jump or scream when they heard they were chosen. They said things like "I've never been happier! My life is gonna change in big ways. I know I'll be smiling a lot more now," "This is the best thing that's ever happened to me," "Everyone knows who I am and they want to hang with me," and "I'm gonna be one of the big people in my school and everyone's gonna want to hang with me and be my friend. It's already started! This is gonna be the best school ever! I love this school!"

Nine of the not-chosen cried during the interview. They made comments like "I hate my life—this sucks! This is the worst!" "What a loser I am," "I just feel so sad ... and so lonely now. I'm never gonna get over this!" "It's like all dirty and disgusting—and that's what I feel inside. I hate this—and I hate me!" and "I don't really like myself anymore. I used to think I was okay but now I found out that I'm not and I just didn't know it." Even though these girls chose to try out, and even though self-chosen competitions are more adaptive than forced competition, in these sorts of high stakes competitions that threaten one's sense of self, the negative emotions can be severe for the losers. The negative effects continued for several months.

Sometimes negative effects are temporary, like for Melanie Wood the mathematician. She participated in the MathCounts Countdown round in which two top-scoring participants sit at buzzers (Olson, 2004). A problem is flashed on the screen that all can see. The two contestants get 45 seconds to hit the buzzer, and then three seconds to answer the question. After a specified number correct, one competitor advances and the other is out. It is intense. Everyone is watching. Melanie Wood said that the Countdown Round was

> the most intense experience I've ever had.... In seventh grade, before my first Countdown Round, I didn't want to do it, but they told me that I had to. So I got up there, and after the very first question I had to run to the bathroom and throw up.
>
> (p. 32)

She does not mention if she came back and won.

Outcomes of competition depend on how the competition is structured (Johnson & Johnson, 2009). According to some experts, competition can be adaptive under conditions of *constructive competition,* which refers to competition that is structured so that winning is relatively unimportant, all participants have a reasonable chance to win, and the rules and criteria for winning are clear. Unfortunately, the experts do not give examples of competition where winning is relatively unimportant (Johnson & Johnson, 2009). They do point out that when winning is very important, negative influences come into play like very high anxiety. There may also be temptation to cheat. There are certainly gradations of the importance of winning; for example, winning or not winning a local science fair makes little difference other than the opportunity to compete at a higher level, while winning a national or international science fair can bring thousands of dollars' worth of scholarships Institutions often attempt to even the playing field so that participants have a reasonable chance to win. That is why high school sports have different divisions for larger and smaller schools. Rules and criteria for winning are usually clear in formal competitions, but rules may change in informal competitions in classrooms or among friends, and those changes can foster bad feelings. In sum, competition can foster motivation under some conditions. Teachers, parents, competition developers, and coaches need to be aware of the better conditions.

Research and Theory into Practice

Response to competition depends somewhat on the gender of the participants. Males may respond more positively than females because males tend to prefer competition compared to females (e.g., Gneezy, Niederle, & Rustichini, 2003). In fact, research with 3- to 18-year-old boys and girls found that both groups *performed* about the same (a math task for older participants and a running task for younger), but there was a 20% difference in *choosing to enter a competitive event*, with males more likely to choose competition (Niederle & Vesterlund, 2011). A review of research concluded that in stereotypical male tasks, when men and women have the same ability, men are more likely to want to compete (Niederle & Vesterlund, 2011, p. 625). "Whereas men are eager to compete, women appear to shy away from competitions" (p. 625). A book on competition (Bronson & Merryman, 2013) concluded that women assess the odds of winning more than men and prefer to compete when they have a chance to win. "It's not that women are naturally risk-averse. They perceive risk quite accurately. It's not that women are afraid of the competition itself, or don't enjoy the competition—it's that they're better at recognizing when they will probably lose" (p. 95). This line of research means that if you use competition in order to foster motivation, you need to consider the gender composition of your group and whether females will be disadvantaged.

The fields of music performance and music education have a long history of competitions. Famous classical musicians such as Martha Argerich (piano), Marcin Dylla (classical guitar), and Vladimir Ashkenazy (piano) have benefited from contest wins. School music programs often require their students to participate in competitions. Studies of high school band competition found that males had more positive attitudes toward competition than females, which fits with research in other domains (Burnsed & Sochinski, 1983). Interestingly, students and parents reported little motivational value in band competitions, but, perhaps in a contradiction, students reported that they liked competing. Administrators, music directors, students and parents did not believe that competitions improved music competence; they endorsed competition because they believed it developed student discipline and created good public relations.

Related to competition is public performance, which refers to situations in which people perform in public, like making a speech, participating in a play, or demonstrating a talent. While there is little formal research on this topic, parents, teachers, and coaches can attest to the power that a public performance has on students' tendency to study and prepare. One study (Bergin et al., 2013) found that when elementary school children were given the opportunity to perform a demonstration of their learning to a school assembly, many of them enthusiastically took it even though they were not compelled to participate. Performing before an audience was more motivating than rewards such as stickers and praise from the principal. Having students make presentations can foster motivation for preparation if the teacher scaffolds preparation.

Case 7.1

As a parent and fan, I have observed many sports events. In some sports like cross-country, track and field, and swimming, I know that some athletes will never win. There may be upsets in team sports, but in individual sports like cross-country, track and field, and swimming, some people never win and probably don't expect to win. They will probably never even place. Yet, they continue practicing and participating. Using motivation concepts from this book such as goal setting, self-efficacy, belongingness, achievement goals, and the good and bad of competition, explain why youth participate in competitions for which they have little or no chance of winning.

Summary

- Competition refers to a situation in which two or more individuals or groups vie for a goal that only one can achieve.
- Competition has been criticized because it can have negative effects like reducing intrinsic motivation, creating excessive focus on winning, fostering cheating, and increasing aggression.

- Research reviews of the effects of competition typically show that competition has negative or neutral effects; on average, competition does not improve performance.
- Competitions can generate motivation, learning, and accomplishments.
- When learners choose to participate in competition, they experience autonomy and generally have a better experience compared to when forced to participate.
- A meta-analysis found that overall, competition was not related to performance because the influence of competition depends on achievement goals. If learners adopt a performance approach goal, they do better than if they adopt a performance avoidance goal.
- Losing a competition can be traumatic while winning can be euphoric.
- Constructive competition refers to competition that is structured so that winning is relatively unimportant, all participants have a reasonable chance to win, and the rules and criteria for winning are clear.

Suggestions for Further Reading

Bronson, P., & Merryman, A. (2013). *Top Dog: The Science of Winning and Losing*. Hachette.

Dutton, J. (2011). *Science Fair Season*. Hyperion.

Kohn, A. (1992). *No Contest: The Case against Competition*. Houghton Mifflin Harcourt.

Olson, S. (2004). *Count Down: Six Kids Vie for Glory at the World's Toughest Math Competition*. Houghton Mifflin.

Chapter 8

How do Diverse Backgrounds Affect Motivation?

The Influence of Socialization, Prejudice, Discrimination, and Multicultural Education on Well-being and Motivation

Cultures and countries vary in how much they value specific talents and what youth are motivated to achieve, such as skill in mathematics or art. Only 24% of US 12th graders scored "proficient" on the 2019 math test of the National Assessment of Educational Progress (National Assessment of Educational Progress, 2019). When students in the US do poorly in math, most parents and teachers shrug it off; they may even say things like "I was never good at math either," as though math competence really doesn't matter (Ripley, 2013). This is less true in other countries such as China, Singapore, and South Korea. In the 2018 PISA international tests of 15-year-olds in 79 countries and regions, the US was below average in math.

While there is wide variation in achievement across countries, the motivation variables that predict achievement are fairly consistent across countries. In a combined analysis of Trends in International Mathematics and Science Study (TIMSS) data and Program for International Student Assessment (PISA) international data, the best non-intelligence predictors of mathematics achievement were self-beliefs such as several different measures of self-efficacy. In addition, the variable "home possessions," which is a measure of socioeconomic status (SES), was a strong predictor. This finding shows the importance of understanding perceptions of competence and SES for understanding academic achievement.

Cultural background influences motivation for which talents are developed, how expertise is taught, and at what age children begin practicing. For example, in China, children learn to make traditional Chinese paintings at a level that seems advanced to Americans. Ordinary Chinese children become very competent at drawing bamboo, goldfish, and roosters, traditional topics of Chinese art (Winner, 1996). Chinese children might seem gifted compared to American children. Similarly, chess is valued more highly in Moscow than in Berlin or Toronto (Charness, Krampe, & Mayr, 1996). Memorizing the Qur'an is common among Muslims in Pakistan and Afghanistan, where there are schools devoted to helping youth memorize, but less so in the US. Talents that are valued in a culture are often introduced at younger ages, and children spend more time practicing them. Members of cultures tend to

DOI: 10.4324/9781003046516-8

adopt the goals of the culture and achieve in domains valued by the culture. As the US becomes increasingly multicultural, it becomes increasingly important for teachers and others in the public sphere to be aware of varied cultures and their values.

Cultural Socialization Practices

Socialization refers to a process by which people learn about their group and how to live in it; socialization communicates group values and motivation. Children are socialized at home and at school. They learn holiday traditions, styles of interaction, musical creations, and artistic inventions of the group. Socialization occurs at different levels, such as within the family, the neighborhood, the ethnic group, and the religious group. Researchers describe several types of socialization, including several types of ethnic-racial socialization. Rather than differentiating ethnicity from race, I follow others in using a metaconstruct in reference to ethnic-racial socialization and ethnic-racial identity (Umaña-Taylor et al., 2014).

Of the several types of ethnic-racial socialization, I focus on *cultural socialization,* which is the process by which youth learn about their ethnic-racial heritage and traditions. "Examples include talking about important historical or cultural figures; exposing children to culturally relevant books, artifacts, music, and stories; celebrating cultural holidays; eating ethnic foods; and encouraging children to use their family's native language" (Hughes et al., 2006, p. 749). Research shows that parents' socialization of their children's ethnic-racial identity facilitates children's knowledge of their cultural background, positive attitudes toward their group, and coping with discrimination (Hughes et al., 2006). In some research, cultural socialization is called *pride and heritage socialization* (Huguley et al., 2019). A meta-analysis found that parental ethnic-racial socialization was significantly associated with child ethnic-racial identity (Huguley et al., 2019). The association was strongest in later adolescence, especially in high school. To the degree that cultural socialization fosters ethnic-racial identity, it is likely to be beneficial for youth. A review of research found ethnic-racial identity is "generally associated with positive psychosocial functioning and mental health outcomes among minority adolescents" (Rivas-Drake et al., 2014, p. 50).

While the existing research on ethnic-racial socialization has generally focused on parent influences, cultural socialization also occurs in schools, sports, and counseling settings. Schools are clearly a place where it is appropriate to talk about historical and cultural figures, expose children to culturally relevant books and other artifacts, celebrate cultural holidays, and encourage native language use. Historically, schools have not done these things well. In fact, in some times and places schools have forbidden the use of native language. In terms of motivation, students are more energized and interested when their own group is woven into the curriculum. The multicultural curriculum is often focused on African American, Latinx, and Asian American, but that focus can be extended. Teachers should consider the specific groups that exist in their classrooms. Latinx often focuses on Mexican heritage, but if the students in a classroom are from Nicaragua, Venezuela, or the Dominican Republic, it may be appropriate to cover events from the Nicaraguan Revolution, the Venezuelan oil economy, or the rapidly growing economy of the Dominican Republic. While teachers may not have the time or autonomy to customize the curriculum, they can insert culturally relevant items as appropriate.

A longitudinal study of 961 African American youth in 17 public schools (Del Toro & Wang, 2021) examined how the adolescents' perceptions of cultural socialization in school predicted their identity exploration and grade point averages over a three-year period. The measure of cultural socialization asked the degree to which students thought the school provided opportunities to connect racial identity with being a good student and the degree to which the school taught about the African American racial group. They found that students who perceived greater school cultural socialization had better grades two years later and experienced greater identity exploration.

When implementing cultural socialization, it is important to recognize that it is not always appropriate for teachers to attempt to teach cultural backgrounds. For example, it might not be appropriate for a non-indigenous person to attempt to teach indigenous culture to indigenous students. A tribal leader explained, "do not teach our children our culture. Use our culture. Use our culture to teach them" (Castagno & Brayboy, 2008, p. 956).

Cultural Capital

Financial capital refers to possessions like money and property that can be invested to gain wealth. *Cultural capital* refers to knowledge and relationships that can be "invested" and used to gain benefits (Lareau & Calarco, 2012). Some educators distinguish cultural capital from social capital, but the concepts overlap, and for simplicity, I will combine them.

Cultural capital can come from teachers. This is important because students with cultural capital tend to have higher achievement than other students (Jæger, 2011). However, the concept of cultural capital can be problematic in the sense that it can suggest a deficit view that lower income kids and families lack knowledge and thinking skills that higher income kids and families have. Therefore, it is important to highlight the strengths, or funds of knowledge, that children from every background bring with them and to avoid a deficit view that emphasizes the abilities and knowledge that learners lack. Instead, emphasize the strengths and background knowledge they bring from their heritage culture. Depending on their backgrounds, students may have extensive knowledge of topics such as agriculture, building trades, engine repair, language dialects, and music. Draw upon their funds of knowledge in ways that attract their interest and highlight areas of competence (Rios-Aguilar et al., 2011).

Nancy Lewis (2017) told of being a sophomore in a Missouri high school and erroneously being put in a Latin class. She considered dropping the class because Latin was for college-bound students, which was not her, but when a friend said Nancy would probably fail Latin, Nancy was motivated by the challenge. So, she enrolled in the class, and over time the teacher directed her into the Latin Club and Latin II. Then the teacher, Miss Hofer, asked what Nancy was doing after high school graduation. Nancy had plans to waitress and maybe go to secretarial school. Miss Hofer said that her grades were good enough to attend Southwest Missouri State and she should. Nancy protested that she could not afford college. Miss Hofer said Nancy could get a work-study job, apply for a tuition scholarship, and live at home. She told Nancy whom to call for advice. Nancy did not. She did not know what to say. Finally, Miss Hofer had Nancy write a script of what to say on the phone. Miss Hofer directed Nancy's motivation. Nancy did as directed, got her parents to agree, and ended up graduating from college and becoming a teacher. Without the cultural capital provided by a concerned teacher, Nancy's life likely would have turned out very differently.

One study found that middle-class parents tended to know teachers, resource specialists, principals, counselors, and special educators because they were friends, relatives, and neighbors. In contrast, working-class parents tended to know construction workers, convenience store cashiers, and factory workers (Lareau, 1989). Learners benefit from cultural capital when they or their families have relationships with people who help them access opportunities (like gifted and talented programs, special summer programs, or internships) or institutions (like universities), share inside knowledge, push them, and give them the confidence to pursue challenging opportunities. Teachers can support students by sharing information and connections that could benefit the students.

Cultural capital and social class go together. Higher income families don't have more motivation; they have motivation for different things than lower income families because higher income families have more access to inside knowledge and friends, neighbors, and relatives with power and influence. Middle- and upper-income parents tend to be better able than lower income parents to help with homework, volunteer at school, and connect with influential people. This supports their children's motivation for school. Research shows that middle-class parents are more likely than lower income parents to try to influence teachers through casual conversation, notes, and phone calls. One middle-class parent said, "I try not to request very often Because if you do that it's like you get ignored. It's better to save your ammunition for 'when you really need it' kind of thing" (Lareau & Calarco, 2012, p. 73). Therefore, teachers should be careful not to be over-influenced by upper income families and under-influenced by lower income families.

A principal wanted to expose her students to university life. She took 31 low-income urban students to visit Vassar College in New York (Lopez, 2016). One of their host professors asked how many of the students planned to attend college. Only two raised their hands; all said they lacked money. The professor explained scholarships, endowments, and how to access money for college. The students were amazed that there might be money for them. They were also amazed at the cafeteria; you just choose the food that you want! After the trip, the students had stronger motivation to attend college and greater self-efficacy that they could. They acquired cultural capital about college attendance that is second nature for many middle-class students. Several years later, two students told the principal that the only reason they went to college was because of the Vassar trip.

Prejudice and Discrimination

Surveys of Black youth show that by age 13, most have experienced racial insults and disrespectful treatment (Martin et al., 2011). Black and Latinx students at a New York City high school reported being followed in stores when they were with their friends and even with their parents; they repeatedly reported being harassed by police officers and experiencing discrimination from teachers (Rosenbloom & Way, 2004). At that school, some teachers were described as uncaring toward Black and Latinx students: "some of the teachers don't care, they don't teach you. I had some problems with teachers, they just passed me, but they did not teach me anything, and that's bad for me, for the state exams" (Rosenbloom & Way, 2004, p. 436). At the same school, a history teacher said that knowing African American history was not important and would not help students. Youth who perceive prejudice and discrimination experience lower motivation in school and less belief that their community will support their personal efforts to flourish.

In order to understand the discrimination that youth experience and its effect on motivation, it is useful to recognize patterns of discrimination. In a review of literature, Benner (2017) stated that compared to Asian American youth, African American and Latino youth are more likely to experience discrimination from adults including in schools, stores, restaurants, and neighborhoods. However, Asian American youth have higher rates of discrimination from their peers in and outside of school. Boys of color experience more discrimination from peers and adults than girls of color.

Children, adolescents, and adults of different ethnic groups who perceive greater racism and discrimination are at greater risk for a long list of negative outcomes such as low academic motivation, depression, low self-esteem, anxiety, illness, and low academic achievement. They are also at greater risk for behavior problems, delinquency, crime, and health risks such as smoking, risky sexual behavior, and substance use (Benner & Kim, 2009; Benner et al., 2018; Martin et al., 2011; Schmitt et al., 2014; Sirin et al., 2015; Stein et al., 2016). Clearly, experiencing discrimination plus related negative outcomes such as depression and low achievement affects motivation. In fact, Benner (2017) reported that "Youth who report greater discrimination tend to struggle more academically and be less prepared for and less motivated to do classwork and homework" (p. 252).

Asian Americans are the fastest growing racial group in the US. They include countries of origin such as India, China, Japan, Bangladesh, Cambodia, and Philippines. Thus, there is much diversity within Asian Americans. Because Asian Americans are often referred to as the model minority, it is sometimes assumed that they do not experience racism or discrimination. In fact, Asian American youth experience slurs and jokes at a relatively high rate compared to other groups of color (Mistry & Kiyama, 2021). At the same time, Asian Americans suffer from being treated as invisible, so it is important that teachers "see" them. In self-descriptions, it is remarkable how many Asian Americans use the word *invisible* or comment that no one *saw* them. For example, a Japanese immigrant woman wrote, "No matter how much I worked, I felt like just a token minority and sometimes even a completely invisible person. I lost my confidence and self-worth" (Yamawaki, 2021, p. 29). One young woman recalled that when she was in high school, "I didn't feel like anyone really recognized me." She felt that even though everyone expected her to have high grades, no one recognized her for her accomplishments: "even though I was co-captain [of the volleyball team] one year, they didn't 'see' me. The school didn't recognize me as the co-captain. They didn't even know" (Chou & Feagin, 2008, pp. 64–65). Asian Americans also suffer from being treated as perpetual outsiders as though they will never be fully accepted into American society and are not "true" Americans (Yip et al., 2021).

Some schools exhibit strife between ethnic groups, which can affect motivation. For example, in a southeastern inner city high school that had a particularly hostile environment, a student reported that "African American students treat Asian American students very differently. I mean, they would make fun of them because of the language that they talk.... And because they can't speak English, other students would talk to them about that" (Mirón & Lauria, 1998, p. 195). Students at a high school in New York City described considerable tension among minority groups (Rosenbloom & Way, 2004). There were tensions and fights between Puerto Rican and Dominican students. "American Born Chinese" (ABCs) were annoyed or outraged when they were confused by others with FOBs (fresh off the boat). Asian American students were consistently harassed by non-Asian American students; this included being slapped, pushed, punched, and mocked.

When conflict among ethnic groups exists, it undermines feelings of belongingness and caring that have been discussed in this book. It undermines desire to attend school. Anxiety about conflict can overwhelm the working memory required to think, remember, and problem solve. In this section, I focus on ethnic-racial prejudice and discrimination but acknowledge that prejudice and discrimination also negatively affect many groups such as women, special education students, religious minorities, and others. Teachers are in a tough position as they attempt to bring together students from varied and sometimes competing backgrounds. Teachers can be effective to the degree that they show the caring behaviors described earlier and include information about varied backgrounds in the curriculum, as described later in this chapter in the section Culturally Responsive Instruction.

Interview: Prejudice Toward Special Education Children

Elementary Special Education Teacher at an Urban Elementary School. Two years of experience

> In my current elementary school I see some discrimination with my students because they are on the autism spectrum. Some students look at them differently and even make comments about how they are different. My response to these students is that "they just learn in a different way." I never hide their autism, but the concept is hard for preschoolers or kindergartners to understand. Even sometimes the teachers turn their backs or move to different parts of the playground when my classroom is sharing the space. It is really disappointing that grown adults have such little acceptance for people, children, who are a little different.

Colorblindness

Many people are proud to claim that they are colorblind and do not see the color of other people's skin. This may seem like an appropriate stance because it seems logical to aspire to treat everyone the same. Claiming to be colorblind allows one to claim an egalitarian stance. However, careful analysis shows that being colorblind can be a problem. Everyone sees skin color, and perceptions of skin color can affect thoughts and behavior. In addition, denying the importance of color can lead to maintaining the status quo and thus maintaining racism. Empirical research supports this analysis. A study of teachers (48% White, 10% Black, 29% Latinx) of immigrant children found that teachers who were high on color-blind racial attitudes tended to have low expectations that their teaching would successfully reach and teach the immigrant students (Cadenas et al., 2021). A study of workers in a large US health-care organization measured Whites' color blindness and multi-culturalism beliefs and the work engagement of workers of color in the same work department. Within departments, Whites who believed in multi-culturalism had colleagues of color who felt relatively engaged at work while Whites who believed in color blindness had colleagues of color who felt less engaged at work (Plaut et al., 2009).

In a review of literature, Plaut and colleagues (2018) reported that people high in color blindness tend to be white, less sensitive to racism, and less understanding of the situations of people of color. People may behave in a colorblind manner intending to foster racially safe spaces for people of color, but people of color often interpret such environments as less welcoming. In contrast, employees of color who work with White peers who espouse multicultural attitudes tend to feel less bias and greater engagement. Overall, the research suggests that in order to engage students and staff of all backgrounds, it is best to avoid color blindness and adopt a multicultural attitude. Teachers and administrators often feel uncomfortable discussing ethnic issues because they fear that such discussions might lead to prejudice, stereotypes, and accusations of racism. Nevertheless, discussions can be positive if they lead to greater understanding and empathy and help rectify inequities. Teachers, therapists, and coaches who talk and behave in a color-blind manner can undermine the motivation of their learners and clients of color.

Microaggressions

One behavior that can reduce motivation is racial microaggressions. Sue and colleagues (2007) wrote that racial microaggressions "are brief, everyday exchanges that send denigrating messages to people of color because they belong to a racial minority group" (p. 273). Examples of microaggressive statements and their perceived meaning include the following:

Table 8.1

Microaggressive statement	Message
"Where were you born?"	You are not American.
"You are a credit to your race."	People of color are generally not as intelligent as Whites.
"You are so articulate."	It is unusual for someone of your race to be intelligent.
Asking an Asian person to help with a math or science problem	All Asians are intelligent and good in math/ sciences.

Microaggressive statement	Message
"When I look at you, I don't see color."	Denying a person of color's racial/ethnic experiences.
A White person clutching their purse or checking their wallet as a person of color approaches	You are a criminal.
"As a woman, I know what you go through as a racial minority."	Your racial oppression is not different than my gender oppression. I can't be racist. I'm like you.
"Everyone can succeed in this society, if they work hard enough."	People of color are lazy and/or incompetent and need to work harder.

From Sue et al., 2007, p. 276

Microaggressions can also demean groups due to gender, religion, sexual orientation, and disabilities. For example, persons with disabilities can experience microaggressions when observers deny the disability experience (We all have some form of disability), ask invasive questions (What happened to you?), try to help when no help is needed (I can do it for you), or make persons with disabilities invisible by ignoring them or avoiding eye contact.

Microaggressions can be offensive and corrosive to the victim and also to observers. People who observe a microaggression can be affected in the same way as the victim.

One measure of microaggressions asks whether other people do the following to you because of your race (adapted from Nadal, 2011):

- assume you are not a "true" American
- treat you like a criminal, act scared of you, or assume you will act aggressively
- hold sexual stereotypes about you
- act as if all people of your race are alike
- suggest that people of your racial background get unfair benefits
- assume you are successful because of affirmative action
- hint that you should work to prove that you are not like other people of your race
- suggest that your racial heritage is dysfunctional or undesirable
- suggest that you assimilate to White culture and downplay your racial background
- treat you like a second-class citizen or ignore you like you are invisible
- dismiss or ignore your contributions because of your race

People who work with children and youth should be aware of microaggressions and avoid them.

Lack of access to relevant reading material can constitute a micro-aggression; a mother said,

> Even though readers and literature are becoming more diverse regarding race and culture, it is very difficult for families to see mixed-race families, families with diverse family formations, or families with disabilities. In the case of my family, we intersect with all three of these identities—and five racial identities. It was a constant search to find readers for my children to supplement their K-12 curricula.
>
> (Steketee et al., 2021, p. 1081)

Tokenism refers to including or pushing forward a person of color to communicate the illusion of inclusivity. A mother said that "We were often asked to include our young Latina daughter's picture in either official school website material or printed pamphlets to advertise the school and school special-education services" (Steketee et al., 2021, p. 1080).

Youth who perceive microaggressions are less motivated to follow educators or leaders who are microaggressive. When environments feel microaggressive, like having few persons of color or little material by persons of color, such as readings and films, the environments undermine the motivation of persons of color. Meanwhile, White observers might not even notice the microaggressions and might wonder why persons of color are angry or avoidant. This description of forms of microaggressions can sensitize you to actions and environmental conditions that communicate devaluing of students and colleagues of color. The authors of a prominent examination of microaggressions (Steketee et al., 2021) recommend the use of a culturally responsive framework, which is the next topic.

Multicultural Education

As educators have attempted to engage varied racial, ethnic, and cultural groups, they have called for approaches such as multicultural education (Banks, 2014), ethnic studies (Dee & Penner, 2017) and culturally responsive pedagogy (Ladson-Billings, 1995). These approaches to instruction highlight the goal of social justice. They emphasize cultural identities. While there are distinctions among the approaches, I will provide a general overview that does not highlight distinctions and will use the term multicultural education. Multicultural education is important for motivation because there are often groups of students who feel alienated and unmotivated because of their group status. They may experience prejudice and discrimination, or they may feel left out because of their religious or other beliefs or because they do not share background experiences. Because of their cultural background, they might avoid common activities like joining a sports team, partying, and dating. The multicultural education literature focuses on racial-ethnic groups, but other groups can also feel like outsiders such as rural students at large universities, religious youth among non-religious or other religions, women in male-dominated domains, persons with disabilities in disability-hostile environments, and so forth.

Instruction that takes into account cultural, racial, and ethnic backgrounds often has two major goals:

1   to introduce all students to varied cultures and experiences, and
2   to recognize the contributions of the heritage cultures of students in the classroom or school in order to improve their well-being and motivation.

These two goals address two problems. First, most students don't know much about the history of other racial-ethnic groups or about the contributions of those groups to the wider culture. Second, members of ethnic-racial groups may seldom see members of their own groups in the curriculum; they benefit from feeling that they are seen and valued, which enhances their feelings of belonging and motivation.

Implementation of goal 2 will depend on the specific cultural heritage. For example, Castagno and Brayboy (2008) asserted that schools and teachers who want to be culturally responsive to Indigenous youth must pay attention to more than cultural background. They agreed that cultural responsiveness for Indigenous youth includes accurate attention to the heritage language and culture of specific tribes, not just "indigenous" in general. Some states have recommendations of how to teach about Indigenous peoples. For example, Michigan has a resource manual to accompany State of Michigan social studies standards (Schellong, 2021).

Examples of Multicultural Approaches

A study by Howard (2001) focused on four elementary teachers who were identified as culturally responsive for African American students. Researchers interviewed 17 of their students to ask how their teachers created an effective learning environment. The attribute they mentioned most frequently was caring, which included things like a pat on the back, stating high expectations for performance, and statements about feelings for the students. For example,

> She is a good teacher because she cares so much about us. She tells us every day [that]she cares, and she puts a lot more effort into the kids who don't want to do it [learn]. She tries to help everybody.
>
> (p. 137)

Recall from the chapter on belongingness that caring teachers communicate care for the students and have high expectations for their performance. Howard's study provides evidence that caring is also a component of cultural responsiveness. In some contexts, caring can also mean being strict and demanding. A 5th-grade student stated that effective teachers need to be strict about students getting their work done. The student said, "If she [the teacher] hollers, it just means she cares about us" (p. 138). In another situation, a 4th-grade teacher became upset with a student for not completing a task. The teacher asserted the student was capable of better work. Later, the teacher had a warm, private exchange of words. The next morning, the teacher found a note that said, "Thank you for being a terrific teacher. Thank you for your toughness. It [the toughness] really got me back on track" (p. 139). Note that not all students found strictness and yelling to be effective.

Two other characteristics of motivating teachers that Howard described were ability to create a classroom community, that is, to "make school seem like home," and to make learning fun. Regarding making learning fun, one student said, "She's funny, and she entertains, and I like when she uses our names in the story" (p. 144).

While a multicultural curriculum can facilitate student motivation and perceptions of teacher caring, it is not as easy to implement as it might seem. Two studies of a multicultural high school reform in a northeastern city (Jacob, 1995; Ulichny, 1996) found considerable tension even after the reform. The school was in a predominantly Hispanic neighborhood and included Dominicans, Blacks, Whites, and students from Cape Verde, Jamaica, Africa, Haiti, Puerto Rico, Laos, China, and others; some were born in the US and others overseas. The curriculum was largely implemented by White teachers who were viewed as catering to the bilingual students. There was conflict over language, with Spanish speakers, who were large in number, saying the most important aspect of their culture was their language, and African American students resenting the speaking of Spanish in the school. African American students perceived the use of Spanish language as exclusionary. They feared that they might be missing important information in class and that Latinx students might be plotting against them in a language they could not understand. The conflict over language also existed in English as a Second Language classes, where Spanish-speaking students outnumbered students from Poland, Syria, and other places (Jacob, 1995). An African-American teacher said,

> There's a large percentage of Hispanic students ... or even students that speak some other language other than English. And most of the Black American students only speak English. And so, they'll be in a class where it will be like, three of them, and 27 people speaking other different languages. And that makes them uncomfortable.
>
> (p. 360)

Despite the emphasis on different cultures, the students continued to seg-regate by ethnicity and culture outside of the classroom, like in the lunchroom. Groups fought over what type of music was played at dances. The Black students reported resenting the Latinx students because they were able to visit their origins in places like the Dominican Republic while the African American students could not trace their origins to specific places in Africa. Latinx students resented the African American students for dominating the school talent show, so they created their own talent show, which angered African American students. This well-meaning pro-gram shows that implementing a multicultural curriculum can be complex.

In an article about multicultural professional development, Parkhouse and colleagues (2019, pp. 436–437) provided a list of changes that teachers made in order to become more culturally sensitive:

- Moved away from thinking that non-White students were deficient.
- Spent more time interacting with individuals and groups in addition to interacting with the whole class.
- Began to notice more inequities within their classrooms or school.
- Learned how to better incorporate students' home cultures and lan-guages and use these as resources.
- Improved in their abilities to teach content areas in culturally respon-sive ways.
- Developed confidence in discussing sensitive topics such as diversity, culture, and poverty.
- Developed confidence in teaching about other cultures.
- Improved their self-efficacy in communicating with culturally diverse students and parents.
- Built positive teacher-student relationships.
- Considered diversity when selecting educational materials.
- Educated students about stereotyping and discrimination.
- Recognized the importance of keeping up with issues related to cul-tural and linguistic diversity.
- Became more aware of their own cultural backgrounds, beliefs, biases, and experiences.

The list can be a checklist for instructors, therapists, and coaches who want to become more culturally sensitive and responsive.

Teachers can bridge cultural borders by engaging students' ethnic culture during instruction. Carol Lee helped African American high school students recognize discourse strategies that they used without overt awareness. The students were in two midwestern urban high schools and averaged very low achievement. She used signifying to teach literary analysis (Lee, 1993). *Sig-nifying* is verbal teasing that uses double meaning and irony, with clever twists and surprises (Smitherman, 2000); it is common in African American cultures. For example, a pregnant woman told her sister, "Yes, I guess I am putting on a little weight." In response, the sister signified on her: "Now look here, girl, we both standing here soaking wet and you still trying to tell me it ain't raining" (Gates, 1988, p. 83). Signifying often has risqué overtones. Signifying is evident in rap and hip-hop music and is part of Twitter communication where tweets can mark Black identity. For example, there are groups that signify on specific Black artists, like this tweet signifying on the R&B singer and rapper Drake:

> @charles_star: I got ride like a bicycle. Huffy. Am I the worlds worst rapper? Puffy. #fakedrakelyrics
>
> (Florini, 2014, p. 227)

Signifying is interpreted figuratively, not literally. Lee asked students to interpret samples of signifying and defend their interpretation. She then asked them to do the same with two novels and a short story set in a Black community that used African American English (*Their Eyes Were Watching God, The Color Purple,* and "My Man Bovanne"). The students learned about irony and figurative language. She taught students to comprehend text more deeply and to problem solve as they analyzed text. Students were motivated and commented that they were not used to thinking so much in school. They performed better on a literary test than students from the same school who had traditional instruction (Lee, 1995).

Teachers who want to engage students intellectually and culturally can ask them to analyze examples of culturally relevant behavior. For example, blackfishing refers to "influencers" on Instagram who "appropriate Black culture and urban aesthetics in an effort to capitalize on Black markets" (Stevens, 2021). Teachers could ask how should one respond if non-Black influencers alter their appearances with dark makeup and Afrocentric hairstyles and make buckets of money from imitating Blackness? Teachers could examine cultural movements like #OscarsSoWhite, related domains like Black Twitter and Latinx Twitter, and media activism (Gutiérrez, 2022). Of course, this would demand effort on the part of teachers to inform themselves and would run the danger of the material not being on proficiency or achievement tests. But it would foster motivation, critical thinking skills, and media literacy.

Some school subjects have more obvious multicultural elements than others. For example, social studies can include slavery, the Civil Rights movement, Japanese internment during WWII, Chinese treatment during transcontinental railroad construction, redlining and lack of access to mortgages for persons of color, the Chinese Exclusion Act of 1882, the lynchings in Los Angeles's Chinatown in 1871, and many other examples. Social studies can also include positive contributions from people of diverse backgrounds. Language arts can expand the canon of literature to include works by persons of color, both in the past and present.

Subjects like mathematics have less obvious paths to cultural relevance. An interview study of mostly White preservice and inservice teachers asked for their views on culturally responsive math instruction. Responses included "mathematics is numbers and does not have anything to do with culture, so while culturally relevant teaching lends nicely to social studies, language arts and the arts, it does not apply in mathematics teaching and learning" (Ukpokodu, 2011, p. 50). Others stated, "Being brutally honest, as a math teacher, I never really thought about the approach to mathematics as needing any diversity. After all, math is universal, the occurrence of uniform and consistent concepts, never changing through time" and "Before taking this course I have never heard of culturally responsive mathematics curriculum" (p. 50).

Nevertheless, mathematics is a subject that needs culturally responsive presentation. Students of color struggle particularly with mathematics and tend not to be motivated to pursue STEM careers that are rewarding and lucrative. Some teachers have made their math curricula more inclusive by doing things like pointing out where mathematical principles were first developed, like in Africa, the Arab world, and the Mayan world. They have pointed out people of color who have participated in important technological advances. They have generated course activities that engage local STEM topics like pollution, representation of persons of color, and population trends.

For example, two teachers in a working-class New York middle school helped students generate data on the topic of overcrowding in their school compared to other schools (Turner & Strawhun, 2004/2005). The unit included measuring spaces, calculating areas, and displaying data. One student said, "[Before] I wouldn't really use math. I would just say, LOOK how much space they have [in their school] instead of what we have [in our school].... But I would really use math now.... Math made my argument make more sense." Students found that their school was overcrowded compared to other schools and requested reform. Students learned about math, data analysis, data presentation, politics of schools, and social justice.

A teacher in a different urban community stated,

> I teach in an urban school and my students are 68% African Americans, 30% Hispanics, and 2% White. In teaching algebraic equations, I begin by using my students' interests. For example, when I make up a math problem I do not just start it out by writing the problem on the board. Instead, I take the students through series of familiar experiences: I ask the class to shout out their favorite hip-hop CDs, the artists and their cultural background and then ask them how

much the CDs cost, the amount of money the artists earn if they sold X number. I also ask them to research the number of artists of their favorite CDs. Then we work together to turn it into some type of algebra problem. Somehow this seems to get more kids engaged in the math than if I would have just put up numbers on the board that don't relate to the kids' interest. (Ukpokodu, 2011, p. 51)

Cultural Aspects of Stories and Literacy

One aspect of cultural background is different notions of what is a good story. Stories can be told orally, such as during story time in elementary school, or they can be written. Teachers may assume that everyone knows how to tell a story, and that the story structure will follow the teacher's expectation. But that is not necessarily true. Within U.S. school culture, stories tend to follow a traditional structure in which the narrator builds a series of events, in chronological order, to a climax and problem solution. Fairy tales like Cinderella follow this structure. However, not all cultures share this conception of story. For example, African American children's stories may weave multiple events into a long, out-of-order account in a way that has been compared to jazz (Bliss & McCabe, 2012; Gardner-Neblett et al., 2012). Their stories may include multiple narratives, vivid imagery, complexity, and rhythmic language in a way that may seem excessively long and disjointed to some teachers. Japanese children's stories may include two or three similar events because multiple-event narratives are considered more interesting (Bliss & McCabe, 2012). Japanese children are taught to be concise in a way that might be considered too sparse by teachers. Speakers from Spanish-speaking communities may emphasize family members:

> These connections between family members and events may sound tangential to some listeners from outside the community but they are in fact an integral part of the narrative experience of the speaker.... [I]n fact, the point of telling a story for Spanish-American narrators may not be to recount events so much as it is to let listeners know about the narrators' families.
>
> (Bliss & McCabe, 2012, p. 134)

The various story formats are not wrong within their cultures, but may be unexpected and considered deficient by some teachers. This can undermine the motivation of students who think that they are producing high quality narratives but receive criticism. If students receive poor responses or low grades for stories that fit their cultural background, they may become discouraged and demotivated.

Students who struggle with school literacy are often motivated to be very precise in their out-of-school literacy, such as in their graffiti and

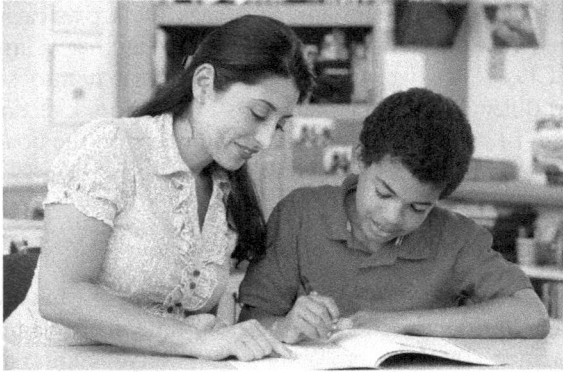

tagging. They may lack motivation for school literacy but are highly motivated in their peer literacy. Moje (2000) wrote that,

> As I watched gang-connected adolescents use literacy, I was intrigued with the contradiction I saw between their motivation to rapidly internalize very specific and complicated gang writing styles, spellings, rules, and dress codes, and their seeming indifference to using conventional writing styles, spellings, punctuation, and grammars.
>
> (p. 652)

For example, Moje observed gang-connected girls who were in Salt Lake City; they wrote notes that followed elaborate rules, such as crossing out the letter O because a rival gang's name began with O (Moje, 2000). These youth engaged in various literacies such as tagging, graffiti writing, hand signs, poetry, and journal writing.

Some youth cross cultural borders, becoming skilled in both in-school and out-of-school literacy. For example, Maria, a Mexican American in Los Angeles, was a tagger (i.e., graffiti writer) and was in AP classes; she said that *The Old Man and the Sea* was a favorite book (MacGillivray & Curwen, 2007). Youth such as these are highly motivated, but not always in the boundaries of traditional school structures.

One way to bridge cultural borders and increase motivation is to use multicultural literature. For example, one Black 4th-grade girl read a collection of poems written by African American authors and then announced, "When I grow up … I want to be a Black poetess" (McGinley & Kamberelis, 1996). A Black 5th-grade boy tried to avoid literacy assignments until he discovered the biography of Fannie Lou Hamer, an African American voting advocate. He became engaged by that book and continued to read biographies about African Americans (Smith, 1995). A Chinese American high school student wrote that reading *The Joy Luck Club* made her proud of her culture (Athanases, 1998).

Students should not read only about their own cultures; a purpose of schooling is to expose students to many different perspectives. A White adolescent read *House of Dies Drear* and was engrossed; she said that when a runaway slave named Thomas dropped his light in a cave, she imagined that she was with him (Spears-Bunton, 1990). Literature helps students understand others who are different (Mar & Oatley, 2008). Thus, students should be exposed to diverse literature as well as to literature that is personally relevant.

Current Events

News events can affect the outlook of students and their motivation in school. In the U.S., attacks on African Americans have caused anxiety for many. In February 2020, Ahmaud Arbery was shot dead while jogging in Georgia. In March, Breonna Taylor was killed in a mistaken police raid. In May, George Floyd was killed by police on the streets of Minneapolis. Nationwide protests erupted amid calls, once again, for reform. There were additional shootings during the period of protests. Students reported feeling anxious and unmotivated for schoolwork.

At the same time, when COVID-19 surged in the US in the spring of 2020, it was reported to have originated in China. In New York City, an Asian woman in her 60s was attacked outside a luxury apartment by a convicted murderer who shouted racial slurs; in Texas, an assailant stabbed three members of an Asian family because he thought they were Chinese and infecting people with coronavirus. In Brooklyn, an Asian woman put out the trash and was splashed with acid that left her with second degree burns. The male assailant ran away. In Paris, five men were arrested for tweeting threatening messages about persons of Chinese ethnicity. When students see these sorts of news events, it can cause anxiety and undermine their motivation for academic work. These are not events teachers can directly influence, but cultural responsiveness calls for schools to respond.

Research and Theory into Practice

In order to understand effects of studying varied groups, one study examined a year-long 9th grade ethnic studies course in the San Francisco Unified School district that resulted in improved motivation. The curriculum covered political struggles of multiple groups and examined

> genocide of American Indians in California; portrayals of Asians, Latinos, and African American in the media; community resistance in historical Chinese and Latino neighborhoods in California; labor

organizing during the Great Depression and World War II among African Americans and Filipino Americans; and social movements and educational reforms contributing to and stemming from the Civil Rights Movement.

(Dee & Penner, 2017, p. 135–136)

The course also included a focus on personal identity, family history, community engagement, and service-learning projects. Researchers found that students in the ethnic studies course increased their attendance by 21%, GPA by 1.4 grade points, and credits earned by 23 (about four courses). The student participants were academically lower achieving with a GPA around 2.0 and were 60% Asian, 23% Latinx, and 6% Black. A follow-up study found that ethnic studies participants continued to have increased attendance in high school, were more likely to graduate from high school, and were more likely to enroll in college (Bonilla et al., 2021). Note that the students in the study started with GPA's around 2.0, fairly low, in 8th grade.

Interview: Prejudice and Discrimination

Elementary Teacher at a Suburban School. One Year of Experience

Growing up as an African American in a school district that was 75.5% white students, 11.2% black students, and 5.4% Hispanic students (DESE District Report), I experienced discrimination throughout my entire K-12 career. There are many different instances I could choose to talk about from growing up as a minority in a district that is so unevenly proportioned, but I want to talk about what it was like as a student teacher. I ended up going back to the district I grew up in to student teach, and I was hopeful that there had been changes made to improve diversity. However, I was very disappointed to find out not much had changed. When I was growing up, in my 13 years in the district, I never had a teacher that was not white. While student teaching, I was the only person of color in my entire school, aside from one high schooler that worked the before-and-after program in the school. In 2020, I didn't expect to be the only person that looked like me in a school. During Black History Month, we were provided with lessons that we were able to teach. There were many problems with the lessons, but the main two were 1) The lessons were about embracing who you are and 2) that even though we are all different, we are all important. While this is a great lesson to teach children, it didn't fit the purpose of Black History Month, which was supposed to be focused on **Black history**. The lessons should have been focused on black history, not about accepting everybody regardless of your skin tone, and it almost had the complete opposite effect that it was intended to. Instead of focusing on black history during the one month dedicated to African Americans, they used it as a time to talk about EVERYBODY which completely missed the point. Like Ta-Nehisi Coates wrote, "Vaguely endorsing a cuddly, feel-good diversity does very little to redress this." The other problem was that some teachers found the lessons "fillers," and I overheard conversations about how pointless the lessons were and how they could be doing more important things If teachers don't think black history is important, I find that very scary. Overhearing conversations like this made me infuriated, but it also made me really sad. Teachers NEED to understand the importance of teaching black history, and realize that part of their privilege is white history being part of the curriculum/being taught all year and black history only being taught as an elective/one month of the year. Next year, I plan on coming up with my own Black History lessons, and I also accepted a job in a different district that aligns more with my values. I know there are other people of color in the building, and the population is much more diverse, so I am looking forward to a change.

When I was a child, during lessons regarding topics like prejudice and discrimination, some students would look at me or would ask my opinion because I was the only person of color in the class, but it never really bothered me. The only instance when I was bothered was when we were learning about slavery in middle school, and a teacher pointed to each African American in the class (there were four of us) and said "If slavery never ended, all of you guys would still be working on plantations." That made me so uncomfortable, and every eye in the room was on us and none of us knew what to say to that.

When I was student teaching, my students were in 3rd grade. Kids are a lot more aware than what we adults give them credit for sometimes, and I was surprised by how much they already knew and how many questions they had. I answered as many questions as I could, but some questions were not for me to answer as an educator in a public school, or they were not age appropriate. So, I told them they could ask grown-ups at home. I had a few kids who told me the next day they asked grown-ups at home. They told me what the grown-ups had said, and it made me really happy to know that I had opened up that conversation and that grown-ups at home were able to continue it.

Case 8.1

Lilia Monzó observed elementary classrooms in a California school that was 99% Latinx and 100% free or reduced-price lunch (Monzó & Rueda, 2009). She noticed that students would claim that they understood English from both the teacher, who spoke only English, and the texts. However, those who had difficulty reading English often mumbled when they had to read aloud. Some said that they did this so that classmates could not detect their mistakes; they also tried to create class disruption that would end their turn of reading. One student, Elizabeth, was very quiet and usually unnoticed by the teacher. On one occasion, after 2.5 hours of supposed essay writing, she had not even written her name on her paper. Monzó said with concern, "Elizabeth, hace dos horas que te estoy mirando y escribiendo lo que estás haciendo, y no has escrito nada. ¿Por qué?" [Elizabeth, I've been watching you for two hours and writing down what you are doing, and you have not written anything. Why?] (pp. 29–30). Elizabeth said that she was going to start, began writing, and mumbled to herself that she did not understand. What concepts from this book help explain the students' behaviors? Why are they pretending to understand when they don't? How do concepts of competence and achievement goals apply?

Summary

- Cultures and countries vary in how much they value specific talents and what youth are motivated to achieve.
- Socialization refers to a process by which people learn about their group and how to live in it; socialization communicates group values and motivation.
- Cultural socialization is the process by which youth learn about their ethnic-racial heritage and traditions.
- *Cultural capital* refers to knowledge and relationships that can be "invested" and used to gain benefits. People with high SES tend to have greater cultural capital.
- Youth of color tend to experience prejudice and discrimination.
- People who experience prejudice and discrimination have higher rates of negative outcomes such as low academic motivation, depression, low self-esteem, anxiety, illness, low academic achievement, behavior problems, delinquency, and health risks such as smoking, risky sexual behavior, and substance use.
- Color blindness can lead to maintaining the status quo and thus maintaining racism.
- Racial microaggressions are brief, everyday exchanges that communicate negative messages to people of color. Microaggressions can also demean groups due to attributes such as gender, religion, sexual orientation, and disabilities.
- Multicultural instruction introduces all students to varied cultures and experiences and recognizes the contributions of the heritage cultures of students in the classroom or school in order to improve well-being and motivation.

Suggestions for Further Reading

DeCuir-Gunby, J. T., & Schutz, P. A. (Eds.). (2016). *Race and Ethnicity in the Study of Motivation in Education*. Routledge.

Gay, G. (2018). *Culturally Responsive Teaching* (3rd ed.). Teachers College Press.

Ladson-Billings, G. (1994). *The Dreamkeepers: Successful Teachers of African American Children* Jossey-Bass.

Chapter 9

How Can You Inspire Motivation in Clients of Counseling, Psychotherapy, Social Work, and Allied Health Professions?

Motivation in the Helping Professions

The principles described in this book apply to widely varied adults who work with youth. That includes parents, coaches, social workers, psychologists, athletic trainers, physical therapists, dieticians, speech language pathologists, health educators, and others. I will refer to this group as interventionists and the people they work with as clients.

A report from the U.S. Surgeon General (US Surgeon General, 2021) described major mental health issues for American children and youth:

> Even before the COVID-19 pandemic, mental health challenges were the leading cause of disability and poor life outcomes in young people, with up to one in five children ages 3 to 17 in the US with a reported mental, emotional, developmental, or behavioral disorder. In 2016, of the 7.7 million children with treatable mental health disorder, about half did not receive adequate treatment.

Unfortunately, in recent years, national surveys of youth have shown major increases in certain mental health symptoms, including depressive symptoms and suicidal ideation. From 2009 to 2019, before the COVID pandemic, the proportion of high school students reporting persistent feelings of sadness or hopelessness increased by 40%; the share seriously considering attempting suicide increased by 36%; and the share creating a suicide plan increased by 44%. Between 2011 and 2015, youth psychiatric visits to emergency departments for depression, anxiety, and behavioral challenges increased by 28%. Between 2007 and 2018, suicide rates among youth ages 10–24 in the US increased by 57%. Tragic early estimates from the National Center for Health Statistics suggest there were more than 6,600 deaths by suicide among the 10–24 age group in 2020.

This distressing report shows that people who work children and youth will face increasing levels of distress and mental health disorders. The report does not once mention motivation, but motivation is key for addressing mental

DOI: 10.4324/9781003046516-9

health and well-being. In this chapter, I will discuss goals, competence, belongingness, autonomy, and cultural backgrounds.

Goals

When clients present, they have goals for seeking intervention, and goals drive motivation. However, with children and youth, the goals may come from the parents or from the children and youth. Sometimes the goals are obvious, but often they are not. The interventionist may have to probe and problem solve to arrive at clear statements of goals. When clients make generic statements like *I want to feel better* or *I want a better relationship*, how to intervene is not obvious. Goals may be apparent in the case of injury situations that require physical or rehabilitation therapy. Even so, there may be hidden or unexamined goals. For example, an injured player may have an obvious goal to get back in competition as soon as possible, or the player may have a non-obvious goal to avoid getting back in competition because the team is a toxic environment or the player fears failing. If the interventionist pushes to get the client back to playing as soon as possible, the client may passively resist, which may surprise the interventionist.

In counseling and social work situations, generating goals is a key aspect of therapy. The concept of approach versus avoidance is an important dimension in goals, which can be described in approach or avoidance terms. "To understand myself and my feelings" is an approach goal while "to stop being confused about my feelings" is an avoidance goal. "To be more confident in social situations" is an approach goal while "to be less shy" is an avoidance goal (Elliot & Church, 2002, p. 245). Recall from the discussion of achievement goals that there are performance approach goals and performance avoidance goals, and avoidance goals tend to have worse outcomes. People who seek therapy often think in terms of avoidance goals because they want to avoid being in stressful work situations, dating the wrong people, gaining weight, and so forth. However, avoidance goals tend to be associated with less change in well-being compared to approach goals (Tryon, 2018). In addition, a problem for interventionists is that avoidance goals provide less information about what is desired than approach goals; avoidance goals tell what to avoid rather than what is wanted (Elliot & Church, 2002). Therefore, it can be useful to frame goals in terms of what is wanted instead of what is not wanted.

Interventionists must collaborate with clients to generate goals. This is more complicated with youth clients because usually the parents are also involved. One study of clinic-referred children (Hawley & Weisz, 2003) examined goals of child, parent, and therapist, that is, what problems they thought should be addressed, and found that about 75% of the triads started treatment without agreeing on even one problem. Therapists tended to agree more with parents than children about child problems.

In the case of very young children or children with cognitive impairments, parents may take a greater role because the child is not cognitively

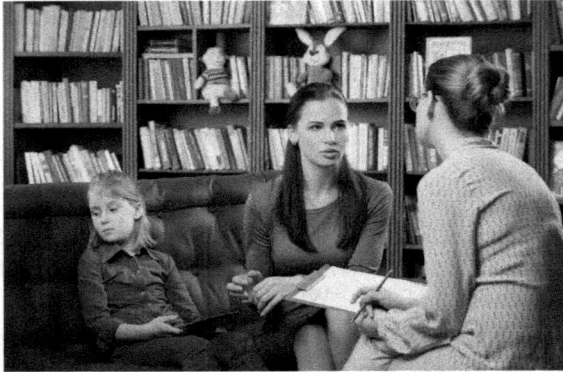

capable of generating and weighing different goals. Ryan (2015), co-developer of self-determination theory, wrote,

> Too often we find ourselves foisting goals on children they may not yet value, understand, or feel able to accomplish. Often, in fact, we don't even ask. Even adults trained in the helping professions are not immune to imposing goals on children as they attempt to act in their "best interests."
>
> (p. 17)

Better collaboration in setting goals is related to greater motivation for therapy. In one study, researchers asked client and therapist to identify the two most important goals in their therapy. They identified the same two goals only 31% of the time, agreed on one of the goals 56% of the time, and did not agree on either goal 13% of the time (Tryon, 2018). A meta-analysis found that psychotherapy outcomes were better when patient and therapist had greater goal consensus and collaboration (Tryon et al., 2018). These patterns suggest that interventionists and clients (children and parents) need good communication and more collaboration than has occurred in the past.

The goal setting process can be effective for interventions. Interventionists often think in terms of SMART goals that are Specific, Measurable, Achievable, Relevant, and Time-bound. Some people refer to the R as realistic instead of relevant. Relevance refers to why the goal is important to the client or what achieving the goal would mean to the client. Chapter 3 gives a more detailed template for effective goals setting that highlights the following: goals are specific, long-term goals are divided into subgoals, goals are challenging, feedback is provided, goal setter is highly committed, goal setter has a plan to overcome barriers, and goal setter shares goal statements with others.

When therapists work on weight issues with clients, evidence suggests that it is best not to set goals that focus on weight (Todd et al., 2015). Focusing on weight can lead to unhealthy thoughts, ineffective dieting, and harm to self-esteem. It is better to focus goals around sensible eating, healthy lifestyle, and behavior change. A healthy lifestyle includes physical activity, and physical activity is not sustainable if the client dislikes the activity. Therefore, it is important to find activities that the client finds enjoyable and sustainable.

Research and Theory into Practice

A study examined the goal setting of 338 male and female athletes in 12 sports who were competing to go the Olympics (Burton et al., 2010). The authors pointed out that most goal research has been set in laboratory settings or used recreational athletes rather than elite athletes; elite athletes have spent a lot of time in their sport and might have a better understanding of goal effectiveness. The authors found that better goal setters had superior athletic performance. The smallest group (38) was termed goal nonbelievers. These athletes had less confidence in the effectiveness of goal setting and lower performance. Note that this study was non-experimental, so it is not clear that the goal setting led to higher performance.

A different study (Gillham & Weiler, 2013) implemented goal setting in a collegiate women's soccer team. They found that the athletes were lackluster goal setters. They set vague goals like "get better," "win," or "improve my dribbling." The coaching staff helped athletes change goals like "score more goals" to "during shooting exercises in practice, 75% of my shots are on the frame of the goal" (p. 100). They eventually achieved buy in from the athletes. They had planned to track individual players' goals, but this turned out to be too labor intensive.

These studies show that using goal setting with athletes is more difficult than might be anticipated, and some athletes will resist. With good support, coaches can get most athletes on board. And they might win more:

> The soccer team finished the season with only the second winning season in the history of the school's women's soccer program.... The positive outcomes from the goal setting intervention were noticed by the starters and seemingly contributed to the increase in team victories for the year.
> (p. 107)

Competence

Self-determination theory claims that humans have an innate need to feel competent. As pointed out in Chapter 3, self-efficacy is a well-studied aspect of competence. Efficacy for change, or the *belief* that you can change, is a key aspect of the ability to change. When clients lack confidence in their capabilities to change, change is less likely. For example, a study (Iannotti et al., 2006) of adolescents with Type 1 diabetes found that self-efficacy for self-management was significantly related to youth following diabetes self-management guidelines for glycemic control; this was especially true of youth who had strong beliefs that adherence would be beneficial. Parents of children with diabetes often experience battles with their diabetic child over self-management, and mothers with high self-efficacy for diabetes management tended to perceive their children (ages 8–17) as having greater self-management skills compared to mothers with less self-efficacy (Leonard et al., 1998). Self-efficacy has been found to be important for adolescents in domains such as diabetes management (Leonard et al., 1998), sexual negotiation (Pearson, 2006), career aspirations (Bandura et al., 2001), physical education (Chase, 2001), substance use (Burleson & Kaminer, 2005), and many others.

Clients' (and interventionists') self-efficacy is influenced by four major experiences. First and usually most important, efficacy is influenced by previous success and failure. Bandura (1997) wrote, "Enactive mastery experiences are the most influential source of efficacy information because they provide the most authentic evidence of whether one can muster whatever it takes to succeed" (p. 80). The young person who fails to lose weight, improve range of motion, or reduce substance use is likely to have lower efficacy than the person who succeeded in the past. Past failure makes future confidence more difficult. A role of the interventionist is to increase efficacy so that change is possible. A review of research in academic settings found that previous mastery experience—success or failure—was the most influential influence on student self-efficacy (Usher & Pajares, 2008). Interventionists can help create situations where children and youth have success, and they can point out times in the past when the clients were successful.

Second, efficacy is influenced by vicarious experience, that is viewing other people succeed or fail. Youth view models, especially their peers, and ask themselves if they can do as well or better (or worse). If they perceive that they are similar to a successful model, they are likely to believe that they can do as well. If they perceive that they are similar to a failing model, they are likely to believe that they will fail. This pattern influences their efficacy to resist peer pressure, to engage in new activities, to engage in sports, to control weight, to avoid substance use, to recover from substance use, and so forth. Interventionists can draw attention to models who would most enhance self-efficacy.

Third, efficacy is influenced by persuasion. When a respected and authoritative person tells a young person that they are capable, their efficacy is likely to be enhanced. At the same time, if a respected and authoritative person tells a young person that they are not capable, it can have long-lasting effects. Such comments could come from a coach who says that an athlete is not likely to be successful, from a substance use counselor who says that an addict is not likely to control their habit, or from a physical therapist who says that a person in rehabilitation is not likely to recover physical ability. Thus, persons in authority should be careful about making negative comments that could negatively affect young people's beliefs about their capabilities.

Fourth, efficacy is influenced by physiological responses. When children and youth get sweaty hands or racing hearts, they can interpret their physiological response as evidence that they lack ability.

Interventionists need to consider what is influencing their clients' perceptions of competence as they work through the counseling process. They can probe why clients believe that they are or are not capable. What experiences gave rise to their beliefs? They can provide competence support through feedback and skill development (Ryan et al., 2011) as well as mastery modeling described in Chapter 3.

Belongingness

Interventions are more effective when people feel connected and cared for. One aspect of connection is therapeutic alliance, which refers to a bond between client and therapist that facilitates therapeutic work. Research with adults has consistently shown a positive relationship between therapeutic alliance and therapy outcomes. A meta-analysis of studies with children and adolescents (Shirk et al., 2011) also showed a positive relationship between therapeutic alliance and therapy outcomes. The meta-analysis is noteworthy because it included only studies that measured alliance prior to outcome, thus showing prediction over time rather than measuring alliance and outcome at the same time.

Interventions with youth are unique because the interventionist must often attempt to establish an alliance with the youth and their parent or parents. This can be even more complicated because often child goals and parent goals are not the same (Hawley & Weisz, 2003).

There are many commentaries on how COVID-19 shutdowns and the use of video for therapy have affected the interventionist-client relationship. Based on anecdotal reports, it is easy to imagine a reduced the bond between interventionist and client. While internet-based video for therapy has improved access for people who must travel long distances for therapy, it has probably reduced levels of warmth with therapists. Nevertheless, a recent meta-analysis of youth psychotherapy delivered remotely—that is, technology-based treatment—found that remote therapies were as effective as those delivered in person (Venturo-Conerly et al., 2022). The psychopathologies that were studied included anxiety-related disorders (including obsessive-compulsive disorder and trauma), depression, ADHD, and conduct-related disorders.

Part of feeling cared for is feeling that others respect your cultural background. This topic is discussed in the diversity section later in this chapter.

Case 9.1

Athletic trainers are in a position where their relationship with the client athlete is crucial. Injured athletes are often in a state of fear and anxiety because they experience doubt about whether they will fully recover, fear that they will reinjure themselves, and loss of identity if they cannot play or even practice (Zakrajsek et al., 2017). In this context, the effective trainer must elicit athlete's trust. One thing that helps trust is that trainers do not generally wield power over athletes. One athletic trainer commented, "And another thing is that we're safe. They tell us everything, probably too much. But we don't determine play, we don't determine scholarship, we don't determine practice, we don't determine anything" (Zakrajsek et al., 2017, p. 224). What can trainers, therapists, and coaches do to foster trust from clients and athletes? What undermines trust?

Autonomy

Ryan and colleagues (2011) pointed out that people do not generally anticipate intrinsic motivation for being in counseling. They do not anticipate that counseling will be enjoyable, interesting, or fun. Rather, they see counseling as instrumental to achieving valued outcomes like improved career, marriage, or health. A key insight is that while seeking counseling might not be intrinsically motivated, it is usually self-determined, autonomous, or self-chosen, and the quality of participation is higher when the degree of self-determination is higher; clients are less distracted during therapy, more satisfied, and have greater intention to persist. Motivational styles relevant to counseling and behavior change can range from amotivation in which a person is pressured into counseling or required to participate in counseling, to integrated regulation in which the person values counseling and feels that seeking counseling fits with personal values and goals, to intrinsic motivation in which the person actually enjoys participating in counseling and the growth that results. Note that amotivation is externally controlled and non-autonomous while integrated regulation and intrinsic motivation are internally controlled and autonomous.

A study at an inpatient unit that treated eating disorders found that providing autonomy supportive informed choice about whether to continue or terminate treatment after a few weeks of treatment reduced the dropout rate (Vandereycken & Vansteenkiste, 2009). In a study that randomly assigned patients to three different types of manualized therapy for major depression

(Zuroff et al., 2012), researchers examined perceptions of autonomy during treatment. They found that clients who felt autonomy support from their therapists (e.g., provides choices and options, explains why) had lower depressive severity compared to clients who felt less autonomy support.

Interview: Therapy with Clients

Social Worker with MSW in an Urban Setting who also does Telehealth. Four years of experience

Social interaction seems to me to be a motivator for kids at school. In my private practice, I have been working with a ten-year-old boy who started therapy because according to his parents, he "just needs someone to talk to" about his issues. The boy displays some anxiety and internalizes things that are not attributable to him, like when a teacher yells at the class and he was not part of the problem but he blames himself. He has always felt pretty negatively about school and has not had many school friends in the past. He is very bright and has good memory when he is interested in things. He spends little time with peers outside of school. Around the time I met him, he switched schools due to parental separation. He spoke negatively about the school and said that he did not like going. However, he slowly started talking more and more about other kids at the school and was clearly making some friends in his classes. When I asked him about school recently, he said that it was "good" and that he "understands topics better." He excitedly described a new concept he was learning in his math class. He is feeling more motivated about his schoolwork and his social interactions.

Another motivator is connection with peers. I started working with another client recently, a 13-year-old female, who speaks negatively about her school. She also switched schools recently due to custody issues with her parents. She said that she did not like her old school and does not like her new school either. She said that she does not talk to other kids in the class because she "doesn't care." There are some girls in her class who sometimes talk to her, but she said that she finds them boring and they "only talk about themselves or school." She said she has had some online friends in the past who stopped talking to her abruptly or told her they didn't like her. Most of her friends in the past have been online. She is not interested in interacting with peers in person and finds it intimidating. She is not doing well in her classes and is on track to fail one this semester.

I worked at a non-profit agency in an urban setting that did group therapy for kids who were referred for behavior issues. They had afterschool programming for ages 11–13. The kids who improved were typically the ones who connected more with staff. It helps if they identify with staff. It seems like if the kid is a young Black male and the staff is a young Black male, there is a greater probability of connection. If the child had a connection with staff, they were more open to listening. Instead of being defensive, they could be logical and understand what the staff were saying. No one wants to listen to someone they don't like. Some staff were more likeable. Some less. The ones who were less would make it apparent when they did not like some children. This was displayed by situations like overreacting to a kid getting a pencil without asking. The less likeable were very power assertive. They would say things like "you have to listen to me because I am the adult and I will take away rewards for the day." Kids might listen to mean staff but would be mad about it and the changes wouldn't last. Rewards staff used included candy for a good day with few behavior issues or an ice cream bar for a really good day. Kids also got tickets for good behavior, up to two a day. When they got 15 tickets, they could pick out of a prize bin with items that included slime, candy, balls, and Takis or other spicy chips. More likeable staff were more laid back, did not overreact, and were generally more calm. They were not necessarily buddy-buddy with the kids, but displayed some warmth and would talk with kids about their day and sometimes joke with them.

What undermines motivation to change? The main influence is their parents. They behave similarly to their parents. The kids with ODD—how do you react to others who annoy you when your parents yell at you and whoop you and hit you? You yell and hit other kids. Another huge thing is external motivation—all the strategies that the parents have for motivation are to hit, yell, and take things away (phone, game consoles, etc.). They do not talk about how they make other people feel, or alternative things they could do in response. The kids learn little about internal motivation at home.

Cultural Background

Research on diversity and cultural background in mental health domains has not typically examined motivation as an outcome variable. However, when people successfully change, one can infer that they were motivated for change. As mentioned earlier, self-determination proponents suggest that autonomous motivation for change leads to higher quality performance than externally controlled motivation for change (Ryan et al., 2011). It is noteworthy that persons of color are less likely to use counseling services than other groups, and when they do start therapy, about half do not show up for a second appointment (Kim, 2010), so paying attention to background characteristics is important for intervention success.

Proponents of cultural competence in therapy argue that therapists' competence to foster change depends on their ability to adapt to the cultural backgrounds of their clients (Sue et al., 2008). For example, some therapies ask clients to share their emotions, but some cultures, such as some Asian cultures, value restraint and discretion; clients may feel motivated to avoid revealing too much (Kim, 2010).

Research to test claims about therapists adapting to cultural background has generally supported adapting. A meta-analysis of culturally adapted mental health interventions found positive effects, though many of the studies were not randomized experiments (Griner & Smith, 2006). This meta-analysis included studies with different age groups and levels of acculturation; it found stronger effects of culturally adapted mental health interventions for less acculturated, often older clients. The authors recommended that interventions be targeted to specific cultural groups and be delivered in the native language, if possible. A second meta-analysis found that when clients reported that therapists were culturally competent, their outcomes tended to be better (Soto et al., 2018). Another review supported tailoring interventions to cultural backgrounds (Huey et al., 2014, p. 315). The authors pointed out that cultural adaptation seems to be more important for older people who are less acculturated compared to children and youth, who are more likely to have adapted to local cultures.

Unfortunately, studies that adapt interventions for cultural background seldom provide detailed descriptions of the adaptations (Soto et al., 2018). Two approaches are obvious—provide therapy in the native language and match the background of the client with the background of the interventionist. More subtle adaptations are not obvious because they are unique and apply to specific cultural backgrounds. Some psychologists have asserted that every therapist should be culturally competent to work with multiple cultures (Sue et al., 2008). Articles assert that interventionists should be sensitive to cultural factors, cultural norms, cultural awareness, etc. but only occasionally give specific guidance. It is important to acknowledge that authors are often hesitant to provide a list of specific accommodations that can be applied to specific cultural groups because it might lead to stereotyping. If articles listed specific language to use and specific topics to avoid based on demographic attributes rather than individual needs, it could lead to inappropriate therapies. In addition, much of the research has been done with adults rather than children and youth. Therefore, interventionists need to be very sensitive to cues provided by child and youth clients and should know something about their cultural background.

Areas in which cultures can differ include the following:

- Meaning of type of dress (casual versus formal) and display of body.
- Meaning of time and punctuality.

- Deferring to people in authority.
- Acknowledging that you don't understand.
- Correcting other people.
- Revealing problems in the family.
- Gender roles such as what is appropriate behavior of males versus females.
- Deferring to older people.
- Eye contact, especially during moments of discipline.
- Meaning of silence.
- Procedure to interrupt during conversation.
- Communicating romantic interest.
- Physical contact like kissing on the cheek and handshakes.
- Physical space during conversations.
- Styles of participation in instructional settings such as students asking questions and stating their opinions.

People are less likely to feel cared for, and therefore less likely to be motivated to follow advice, if they feel that their culture is ignored or maligned. They may not even recognize the reason for their lack of motivation; they just feel as though the advice does not apply to them or fit their needs. In an interview study (Muñoz, 2007), occupational therapists who were culturally responsive described their experiences providing occupational therapy to diverse populations. They said that therapists needed to build cultural awareness. One therapist said she needed to find out

> What do people do? How do they do it? How do they go about it? How does their cultural group do things? How do they deal with sickness and health and things like this? And even the mundane things of eating, sitting, toileting and such? … I find out some of this by reading, but a lot more by asking the people I treat.
>
> (p. 267)

A relevant question the interventionist can ask is "As we are working in therapy, you need to let me know if we are doing anything that doesn't feel right for you or goes against your culture" (p. 269).

Conclusion

Some people seem to think that kids either have motivation or they don't. Research cited in this book shows that teachers, parents, therapists, and coaches have a lot of influence on youth motivation. Some people think that the way to motivate youth is through pressure and extrinsic rewards. Research cited in this book shows that pressure and extrinsic rewards are usually ineffective in the long term. I hope that this book has convinced you that you can influence motivation but should not attempt to control it.

If you support goals, perceptions of competence, belongingness, autonomy, and meaningfulness, you will go a long way toward supporting motivation. At the same time, you could consider whether competition would foster or thwart development of adaptive motivation in the situations that you face. And always consider the background culture of learners.

Summary

- The principles described in this book apply to widely varied adults who work with youth. That includes parents, coaches, social workers, psychologists, athletic trainers, physical therapists, dieticians, speech language pathologists, health educators, and others.
- Goals are key for designing interventions. The interventionist may have to probe and problem solve to arrive at clear statements of goals.
- Self-efficacy, a key concept of competence, is essential for motivation for change. When clients or interventionists lack efficacy for change, change is less likely.
- The need for belongingness influences intervention outcomes.
- The therapeutic alliance refers to a bond between client and therapist that facilitates therapeutic work. Interventions with youth are unique because the interventionist must often attempt to establish an alliance with the youth and their parent or parents.
- While seeking counseling might not be intrinsically motivated it is usually self-determined, and the quality of participation is higher when the degree of self-determination is higher; clients are less distracted during therapy, more satisfied, and have greater intention to persist.

References

Abernathy, T. V., & Vineyard, R. N. (2001). Academic competitions in science: What are the rewards for students? *The Clearing House*, 74(5), 269–276.

Adams, M. J. (1990). *Beginning to Read: Thinking and Learning about Print. A Summary.* University of Illinois.

Alexander, P. A., Jetton, T. L., & Kulikowich, J. M. (1995). Interrelationship of knowledge, interest, and recall: Assessing a model of domain learning. *Journal of Educational Psychology*, 87(4), 559–575.

Alexander, P. A., Schallert, D. L., & Reynolds, R. E. (2009). What is learning anyway? A topographical perspective considered. *Educational Psychologist*, 44(3), 176–192.

Alexanderson, G. L., Klosinski, L. F., & Larson, L. C. (Eds.). (1985). *The William Lowell Putnam Mathematical Competition Problems and Solutions.* The Mathematical Association of America.

Anderman, E., & Wolters, C. (2006). Goals, values, and affect: Influences on student motivation. In P. Alexander & P. Winne (Eds.), *Handbook of Educational Psychology* (2nd ed., pp. 369–389). Erlbaum.

Ariely, D., Gneezy, U., Loewenstein, G., & Mazar, N. (2009). Large stakes and big mistakes. *The Review of Economic Studies*, 76(2), 451–469.

Assor, A., Kaplan, H., Kanat-Maymon, Y., & Roth, G. (2005). Directly controlling teacher behaviors as predictors of poor motivation and engagement in girls and boys: The role of anger and anxiety. *Learning and Instruction*, 15(5), 397–413.

Assor, A., Kaplan, H., & Roth, G. (2002). Choice is good, but relevance is excellent: Autonomy-enhancing and suppressing teacher behaviours predicting students' engagement in schoolwork. *British Journal of Educational Psychology*, 72(2), 261–278.

Athanases, S. Z. (1998). Diverse learners, diverse texts: Exploring identity and difference through literary encounters. *Journal of Literacy Research*, 30(2), 273–296.

Atwell, N. (2015, April 16). The 'most powerful' classroom innovation–by the $1 million teaching prize winner. *Washington Post*.

Autin, F., & Croizet, J.-C. (2012). Improving working memory efficiency by reframing metacognitive interpretation of task difficulty. *Journal of Experimental Psychology: General*, 141(4), 610–618.

Bae, C. L., Mills, D. C., Zhang, F., Sealy, M., Cabrera, L., & Sea, M. (2021). A systematic review of science discourse in K–12 urban classrooms in the United

States: Accounting for individual, collective, and contextual factors. *Review of Educational Research,* 91(6), 831–877.

Bandura, A. (1997). *Self-efficacy: The Exercise of Control.* Freeman.

Bandura, A. (2012). On the functional properties of perceived self-efficacy revisited. *Journal of Management,* 38(1), 9–44.

Bandura, A., Barbaranelli, C., Caprara, G. V., & Pastorelli, C. (2001). Self-efficacy beliefs as shapers of children's aspirations and career trajectories. *Child Development,* 72(1), 187–206.

Banks, J. A. (2014). *An Introduction to Multicultural Education* (5th ed.). Pearson.

Barber, B. K., Xia, M., Olsen, J. A., McNeely, C. A., & Bose, K. (2012). Feeling disrespected by parents: Refining the measurement and understanding of psychological control. *Journal of Adolescence,* 35(2), 273–287.

Barnett, L. A. (2006). Flying high or crashing down: Girls' accounts of trying out for cheerleading and dance. *Journal of Adolescent Research,* 21(5), 514–541.

Barnett, L. A. (2007). 'Winners' and "losers": The effects of being allowed or denied entry into competitive extracurricular activities. *Journal of Leisure Research,* 39(2), 316–344.

Baumeister, R. F., & Leary, M. R. (1995). The need to belong: Desire for interpersonal attachments as a fundamental human motivation. *Psychological Bulletin,* 117, 497–529.

Behnke, A. O., Piercy, K. W., & Diversi, M. (2004). Educational and occupational aspirations of Latino youth and their parents. *Hispanic Journal of Behavioral Sciences,* 26(1), 16–35.

Beilock, S. L. (2008). Math performance in stressful situations. *Current Directions in Psychological Science,* 17(5), 339–343.

Beilock, S. L., Gunderson, E. A., Ramirez, G., & Levine, S. C. (2010). Female teachers' math anxiety affects girls' math achievement. *Proceedings of the National Academy of Sciences,* 107(5), 1860–1863.

Benner, A. (2017). The toll of racial/ethnic discrimination on adolescents' adjustment. *Child Development Perspectives,* 11(4), 251–256.

Benner, A. D., & Kim, S. Y. (2009). Experiences of discrimination among Chinese American adolescents and the consequences for socioemotional and academic development. *Developmental Psychology,* 45(6), 1682–1694.

Benner, A. D., Wang, Y., Shen, Y., Boyle, A. E., Polk, R., & Cheng, Y.-P. (2018). Racial/ethnic discrimination and well-being during adolescence: A meta-analytic review. *American Psychologist,* 73(7), 855–883.

Bergin, C., & Bergin, D. A. (2009). Attachment in the classroom. *Educational Psychology Review,* 21(2), 141–170.

Bergin, D. A. (1999). Influences on classroom interest. *Educational Psychologist,* 34(2), 87–98.

Bergin, D. A. (2016). Social influences on interest. *Educational Psychologist,* 51(1), 7–22.

Bergin, D. A., & Cooks, H. C. (2000). Academic competition among students of color: An interview study. *Urban Education,* 35(4), 442–472.

Bergin, D. A., & Prewett, S. (2020). Goal concepts for understanding and improving the performance of students with learning disabilities. In A. Martin, R. Sperling, & K. Newton (Eds.), *Handbook of Educational Psychology and Students with Special Needs* (pp. 315–338). Routledge.

Bergin, D. A., Cooks, H. C., & Bergin, C. C. (2007). Effects of a college access program for youth underrepresented in higher education: A randomized experiment. *Research in Higher Education*, 48(6), 727–750.

Bergin, D. A., Bergin, C., Van Dover, T., & Murphy, B. (2013). Learn more: Show what you know. *Phi Delta Kappan*, 95(1), 54–60.

Bergner, D. (2016). *Sing for Your Life: A Story of Race, Music, and Family*. Little, Brown and Company.

Bess, S. (1994). *Nobody Don't Love Nobody*. Gold Leaf Press.

Beymer, P. N., Rosenberg, J. M., & Schmidt, J. A. (2020). Does choice matter or is it all about interest? An investigation using an experience sampling approach in high school science classrooms. *Learning and Individual Differences*, 78, 101812.

Bian, L., Leslie, S.-J., Murphy, M. C., & Cimpian, A. (2018). Messages about brilliance undermine women's interest in educational and professional opportunities. *Journal of Experimental Social Psychology*, 76, 404–420.

Binder, A. J., & Abel, A. R. (2018). Symbolically maintained inequality: How Harvard and Stanford students construct boundaries among elite universities. *Sociology of Education*, 92(1), 41–58.

Binning, K., Wang, M.-T., & Amemiya, J. (2019). Persistence mindset among adolescents: Who benefits from the message that academic struggles are normal and temporary? *Journal of Youth and Adolescence*, 48(2), 269–286.

Birchwood, D., Roberts, K., & Pollock, G. (2008). Explaining differences in sport participation rates among young adults: Evidence from the South Caucasus. *European Physical Education Review*, 14(3), 283–298.

Bishop, J. H., Bishop, M., Bishop, M., Gelbwasser, L., Green, S., Peterson, E., Rubinsztaj, A., & Zuckerman, A. (2004). Why we harass nerds and freaks: A formal theory of student culture and norms. *Journal of School Health*, 74(7), 235–251.

Bishop, K., & Walters, H. (2007). The National Ocean Sciences Bowl: Extending the reach of a high school academic competition to college, careers, and a lifelong commitment to science. *American Secondary Education*, 35(3), 63–76.

Blackwell, L. S., Trzesniewski, K. H., & Dweck, C. S. (2007). Implicit theories of intelligence predict achievement across an adolescent transition: A longitudinal study and an intervention. *Child Development*, 78(1), 246–263.

Bliss, L., & McCabe, A. (2012). Personal narratives: Assessment and intervention. *Perspectives on Language Learning and Education*, 19(4), 130–138.

Blumenfeld, P. C., & Meece, J. L. (1988). Task factors, teacher behavior, and students' involvement and use of learning strategies in science. *Elementary School Journal*, 88(3), 235–250.

Boaler, J. (2008). *What's Math Got To Do With It?* Viking.

Bonilla, S., Dee, T. S., & Penner, E. K. (2021). Ethnic studies increases longer-run academic engagement and attainment. *Proceedings of the National Academy of Sciences*, 118(37), e2026386118.

Brassell, D. (2017). A change in strategy. In A. Newmark & A. Kajitani (Eds.), *Inspiration for Teachers* (pp. 158–161). Chicken Soup for the Soul.

Breakstone, J., Smith, M., Wineburg, S., Rapaport, A., Carle, J., Garland, M., & Saavedra, A. (2021). Students' civic online reasoning: A national portrait. *Educational Researcher*, 50(8), 505–515.

Bronson, P., & Merryman, A. (2013). *Top Dog: The Science of Winning and Losing*. Hachette.

Brooks, A. W. (2014). Get excited: Reappraising pre-performance anxiety as excitement. *Journal of Experimental Psychology: General*, 143(3), 1144–1158.

Brown, M., Brown, P., & Bibby, T. (2008). "I would rather die": Reasons given by 16-year-olds for not continuing their study of mathematics. *Research in Mathematics Education*, 10(1), 3–18.

Bryan, A. D., Aiken, L. S., & West, S. G. (1996). Increasing condom use: Evaluation of a theory-based intervention to prevent sexually transmitted diseases in young women. *Health Psychology*, 15(5), 371–382.

Buentello, J. (2017). The smallest sign. In A. Newmark & A. Kajitani (Eds.), *Inspiration for Teachers* (pp. 339–341). Chicken Soup for the Soul.

Burleson, J. A., & Kaminer, Y. (2005). Self-efficacy as a predictor of treatment outcome in adolescent substance use disorders. *Addictive Behaviors*, 30(9), 1751–1764.

Burnsed, V., & Sochinski, J. (1983). Research on competitions: Surveys reveal how students, parents, directors, and administrators feel about competitions. *Music Educators Journal*, 70(2), 25–27.

Burton, D., Pickering, M., Weinberg, R., Yukelson, D., & Weigand, D. (2010). The competitive goal effectiveness paradox revisited: Examining the goal practices of prospective Olympic athletes. *Journal of Applied Sport Psychology*, 22(1), 72–86.

Cadenas, G. A., Cisneros, J., Spanierman, L. B., Yi, J., & Todd, N. R. (2021). Detrimental effects of color-blind racial attitudes in preparing a culturally responsive teaching workforce for immigrants. *Journal of Career Development*, 48(6), 1–16.

Calderwood, C., Ackerman, P. L., & Conklin, E. M. (2014). What else do college students "do" while studying? An investigation of multitasking. *Computers & Education*, 75, 19–29.

Campbell, J. R., & Walberg, H. J. (2010). Olympiad studies: Competitions provide alternatives to developing talents that serve national interests. *Roeper Review*, 33(1), 8–17.

Canning, E. A., & Harackiewicz, J. M. (2015). Teach it, don't preach it: The differential effects of directly-communicated and self-generated utility–value information. *Motivation Science*, 47–71.

Castagno, A. E., & Brayboy, B. M. J. (2008). Culturally responsive schooling for indigenous youth: A review of the literature. *Review of Educational Research*, 78 (4), 941–993.

Chase, M. A. (2001). Children's self-efficacy, motivational intentions, and attributions in physical education and sport. *Research Quarterly for Exercise and Sport*, 72(1), 47–54.

Chen, P., Chavez, O., Ong, D. C., & Gunderson, B. (2017). Strategic resource use for learning: A self-administered intervention that guides self-reflection on effective resource use enhances academic performance. *Psychological Science*, 28(6), 774–785.

Chen, P., Powers, J. T., Katragadda, K. R., Cohen, G. L., & Dweck, C. S. (2020). A strategic mindset: An orientation toward strategic behavior during goal pursuit. *Proceedings of the National Academy of Sciences*, 117(25), 14066.

Chesley, L. (1973). *Seven Years in Hanoi*. Bookcraft.

Chou, R., & Feagin, J. (2008). *The Myth of the Model Minority*. Paradigm.

Chutel, L., & Kazeem, Y. (2018). Marvel's 'Black Panther' is a broad mix of African cultures—here are some of them. Retrieved from https://qz.com/africa/1210704/black-panthers-african-cultures-and-influences/

Cialdini, R. B. (2005). What's the best secret device for engaging student interest? The answer is in the title. *Journal of Social and Clinical Psychology*, 24(1), 22–29.

Cisneros, S. (2015). *A House of My Own*. Knopf.

Cooper, K., & Miness, A. (2014). The co-creation of caring student-teacher relationships: Does teacher understanding matter? *The High School Journal*, 97(4), 264–290.

Cordova, D. I., & Lepper, M. R. (1996). Intrinsic motivation and the process of learning: Beneficial effects of contextualization, personalization, and choice. *Journal of Educational Psychology*, 88(4), 715–730.

Czerski, H. (2017). The fascinating physics of everyday life [TED talk]. Retrieved from www.youtube.com/watch?v=_ryJK294Psw&t=527s

Darner, R. (2019). How can educators confront science denial? *Educational Researcher*, 48(4), 229–238.

Deci, E. L., & Ryan, R. M. (Eds.). (2002). *Handbook of Self-Determination Research*. University of Rochester Press.

Dee, T. S., & Penner, E. K. (2017). The causal effects of cultural relevance. *American Educational Research Journal*, 54(1), 127–166.

Del Toro, J., & Wang, M.-T. (2021). School cultural socialization and academic performance: Examining ethnic-racial identity development as a mediator among African American adolescents. *Child Development*, 92(4), 1458–1475.

Diethelm, P., & McKee, M. (2009). Denialism: What is it and how should scientists respond? *European Journal of Public Health*, 19(1), 2–4.

diSessa, A. (2000). *Changing Minds*. MIT Press.

Done, P. (2005). *32 Third Graders and One Class Bunny*. Touchstone.

Dutton, J. (2011). *Science Fair Season*. Hyperion.

Dweck, C. S. (1986). Motivational processes affecting learning. *American Psychologist*, 41(10), 1040–1048.

Dweck, C. S. (2010). Even geniuses work hard. *Educational Leadership*, 68(1), 16–20.

Dweck, C. S., & Yeager, D. S. (2019). Mindsets: A view from two eras. *Perspectives on Psychological Science*, 14(3), 481–496.

Ehret, C. (2018). Moments of teaching and learning in a children's hospital: Affects, textures, and temporalities. *Anthropology & Education Quarterly*, 49(1), 53–71.

Elliot, A. J., & Church, M. A. (2002). Client articulated avoidance goals in the therapy context. *Journal of Counseling Psychology*, 49(2), 243–254.

Emdin, C. (2016). *For White Folks who Teach in the Hood … And the Rest of Y'all Too: Reality Pedagogy and Urban Education*. Beacon.

Epstein, D. (2013). *The Sports Gene*. Penguin.

Epstein, J. A., & Harackiewicz, J. M. (1992). Winning is not enough: The effects of competition and achievement orientation on intrinsic interest. *Personality and Social Psychology Bulletin*, 18(2), 128–138.

Epton, T., Currie, S., & Armitage, C. J. (2017). Unique effects of setting goals on behavior change: Systematic review and meta-analysis. *Journal of Consulting and Clinical Psychology*, 85(12), 1182–1198.

Ericsson, K. A. (2021). Given that the detailed original criteria for deliberate practice have not changed, could the understanding of this complex concept have improved over time? A response to Macnamara and Hambrick (2020). *Psychological Research*, 85(3) 1114–1120.

Ericsson, K. A., & Pool, R. (2016). *Peak: Secrets from the New Science of Expertise.* Mariner Books.

Estes, T. (2017). History in our heads. In A. Newmark & A. Kajitani (Eds.), *Inspiration for Teachers* (pp. 201–203). Chicken Soup for the Soul.

Falk, J. H., & Adelman, L. M. (2003). Investigating the impact of prior knowledge and interest on aquarium visitor learning. *Journal of Research in Science Teaching*, 40(2), 163–176.

Fast, L. A., Lewis, J. L., Bryant, M. J., Bocian, K. A., Cardullo, R. A., Rettig, M., & Hammond, K. A. (2010). Does math self-efficacy mediate the effect of the perceived classroom environment on standardized math test performance? *Journal of Educational Psychology*, 102(3), 729–740.

Flink, D. (2014). *Thinking Differently.* HarperCollins.

Florini, S. (2014). Tweets, tweeps, and signifyin': Communication and cultural performance on "Black Twitter". *Television & New Media*, 15(3), 223–237.

Ford, M., & Nichols, C. (1991). Using goal assessments to identify motivational patterns and facilitate behavioral regulation and achievement. In M. L. Maehr & P. R. Pintrich (Eds.), *Advances in Motivation and Achievement.* (Vol. 7, pp. 51–84). JAI.

Frey, D. (1994). *The Last Shot.* Houghton Mifflin.

Fryer, R. G. (2010). *Financial Incentives and Student Achievement: Evidence from Randomized Trials.* Unpublished manuscript, Harvard University.

Fryer, R. G., Jr. (2011). Financial incentives and student achievement: Evidence from randomized trials. *The Quarterly Journal of Economics*, 126(4), 1755–1798.

Gardner-Neblett, N., Pungello, E. P., & Iruka, I. U. (2012). Oral narrative skills: Implications for the reading development of African American children. *Child Development Perspectives*, 6(3), 218–224.

Garner, R., Gillingham, M. G., & White, C. S. (1989). Effects of "seductive details" on macroprocessing and microprocessing in adults and children. *Cognition and Instruction*, 6(1), 41–57.

Gates, H. L. (1988). *The Signifying Monkey: A Theory of Afro-American Literary Criticism.* Oxford.

Gillham, A., & Weiler, D. (2013). Goal setting with a college soccer team: What went right, and less-than-right. *Journal of Sport Psychology in Action*, 4(2), 97–108.

Girod, M., & Wong, D. (2002). An aesthetic (Deweyan) perspective on science learning: Case studies of three fourth graders. *The Elementary School Journal*, 102(3), 199–224.

Gneezy, U., Niederle, M., & Rustichini, A. (2003). Performance in competitive environments: Gender differences. *Quarterly Journal of Economics*, 118(3), 1049–1074.

Gollwitzer, P. M., & Oettingen, G. (2012). Goal pursuit. In R. M. Ryan (Ed.), *The Oxford Handbook of Human Motivation* (pp. 208–231). Oxford.

Gollwitzer, P. M., & Sheeran, P. (2006). Implementation intentions and goal achievement: A meta-analysis of effects and processes. *Advances in Experimental Social Psychology*, 38(6), 69–119.

Gorney, R., & Long, J. M. (1980). Cultural determinants of achievement, aggression, and psychological distress. *Archives of General Psychiatry*, 37(4), 452–459.

Green, E. (2014, July 23). Why do Americans stink at math? *The New York Times Magazine*. Retrieved from www.nytimes.com/2014/07/27/magazine/why-do-americans-stink-at-math.html

Greene, R. (2008). Kids do well if they can. *Phi Delta Kappan*, 90(3), 160–167.

Greene, R. (2010). Calling all frequent fliers. *Educational Leadership*, 68(2), 28–34.

Gregory, A., & Weinstein, R. S. (2008). The discipline gap and African Americans: Defiance or cooperation in the high school classroom. *Journal of School Psychology*, 46(4), 455–475.

Gresham, G. (2018). Preservice to inservice: Does mathematics anxiety change with teaching experience? *Journal of Teacher Education*, 69(1), 90–107.

Griner, D., & Smith, T. B. (2006). Culturally adapted mental health intervention: A meta-analytic review. *Psychotherapy*, 43(4), 531–548.

Groendes, L. (2017). When the going gets tough. In A. Newmark & A. Kajitani (Eds.), *Inspiration for Teachers* (pp. 189–191). Chicken Soup for the Soul.

Gunderson, E., Ramirez, G., Levine, S., & Beilock, S. (2012). The role of parents and teachers in the development of gender-related math attitudes. *Sex Roles*, 66 (3–4), 153–166.

Gutiérrez, A. (2022). Situating representation as a form of erasure: #OscarsSoWhite, Black Twitter, and Latinx Twitter. *Television & New Media*, 23(1), 100–118.

Hagenauer, G., & Volet, S. E. (2014). Teacher–student relationship at university: An important yet under-researched field. *Oxford Review of Education*, 40(3), 370–388.

Hattie, J. (2009). *Visible Learning: A Synthesis of over 800 Meta-Analyses Relating to Achievement*. Routledge.

Hawley, K., & Weisz, J. (2003). Child, parent and therapist (dis)agreement on target problems in outpatient therapy: The therapist's dilemma and its implications. *Journal of Consulting and Clinical Psychology*, 71(1), 62–70.

Hayoz, C., Klostermann, C., Schmid, J., Schlesinger, T., & Nagel, S. (2017). Intergenerational transfer of a sports-related lifestyle within the family. *International Review for the Sociology of Sport*, 54(2), 182–198.

Heddy, B. C., & Pugh, K. J. (2015). Bigger is not always better: Should educators aim for big transformative learning events or small transformative experiences? *Journal of Transformative Learning*, 3(1), 52–58.

Helmreich, R. L., Spence, J. T., Beane, W. E., Lucker, G. W., & Matthews, K. A. (1980). Making it in academic psychology: Demographic and personality correlates of attainment. *Journal of Personality and Social Psychology*, 39(5), 896–908.

Henderlong, J., & Lepper, M. R. (2002). The effects of praise on children's intrinsic motivation: A review and synthesis. *Psychological Bulletin*, 128(5), 774–795.

Hilliard, M. E., Powell, P. W., & Anderson, B. J. (2016). Evidence-based behavioral interventions to promote diabetes management in children, adolescents, and families. *American Psychologist*, 71(7), 590–601.

Hirsch, J. L., & Clark, M. S. (2018). Multiple paths to belonging that we should study together. *Perspectives on Psychological Science*, 14(2), 238–255.

Howard, T. C. (2001). Telling their side of the story: African-American students' perceptions of culturally relevant teaching. *The Urban Review*, 33(2), 131–149.

Huey, S. J., Tilley, J. L., Jones, E O., & Smith, C. A. (2014). The contribution of cultural competence to evidence-based care for ethnically diverse populations. *Annual Review of Clinical Psychology*, 10(1), 305–338.

Hughes, D., Rodriguez, J., Smith, E. P., Johnson, D. J., Stevenson, H. C., & Spicer, P. (2006). Parents' ethnic-racial socialization practices: A review of research and directions for future study. *Developmental Psychology*, 42(5), 747–770.

Huguley, J. P., Wang, M.-T., Vasquez, A. C., & Guo, J. (2019). Parental ethnic–racial socialization practices and the construction of children of color's ethnic–racial identity: A research synthesis and meta-analysis. *Psychological Bulletin*, 145(5), 437–458.

Hulbert, A. (2018). *Off the Charts: The Hidden Lives and Lessons of American Child Prodigies*. Knopf.

Hulleman, C. S., & Harackiewicz, J. M. (2021). The utility-value intervention. In G. Walton & A. Crum (Eds.), *Handbook of Wise Interventions* (pp. 100–125). Guilford.

Iannotti, R. J., Schneider, S., Nansel, T. R., Haynie, D. L., Plotnick, L. P., Clark, L. M., Sobel, D. O., & Simons-Morton, B. (2006). Self-efficacy, outcome expectations, and diabetes self-management in adolescents with Type 1 diabetes. *Journal of Developmental & Behavioral Pediatrics*, 27(2).

Isaacson, W. (2021). *The Code Breaker*. Simon & Schuster.

Iyengar, S. S., & Lepper, M. R. (1999). Rethinking the value of choice: A cultural perspective on intrinsic motivation. *Journal of Personality and Social Psychology*, 76(3), 349–366.

Jacob, B. A. (1995). Defining culture in a multicultural environment: An ethnography of Heritage High School. *American Journal of Education*, 103, 339–376.

Jæger, M. M. (2011). Does cultural capital really affect academic achievement? New evidence from combined sibling and panel data. *Sociology of Education*, 84(4), 281–298.

Jamieson, J. P., Mendes, W. B., Blackstock, E., & Schmader, T. (2010). Turning the knots in your stomach into bows: Reappraising arousal improves performance on the GRE. *Journal of Experimental Social Psychology*, 46(1), 208–212.

Jeffrey, A., Auger, R., & Pepperell, J. (2013). If we're ever in trouble they're always there: A qualitative study of teacher-student caring. *The Elementary School Journal*, 114(1), 100–117.

Johnson, D. W., & Johnson, R. T. (2009). An educational psychology success story: Social interdependence theory and cooperative learning. *Educational Researcher*, 38(5), 365–379.

Johnson, D. W., Maruyama, G., Johnson, R. T., Nelson, D., & Skon, L. (1981). Effects of cooperative, competitive, and individualistic goal structures on achievement: A meta-analysis. *Psychological Bulletin*, 89(1), 47–62.

Kamii, C. (1989). *Double-Column Addition: A Teacher Uses Piaget's Theory* [VHS videotape]. New York: Teachers College Press.

Katz, I., & Assor, A. (2007). When choice motivates and when it does not. *Educational Psychology Review*, 19(4), 429–442.

Kelsey, B. (2016). Get your butt in the gym. Big Ten Network. Retrieved from www.youtube.com/watch?v=TcxjQtFUvTA&ab_channel=BigTenNetwork

Kenny, D. (2012). *Born to Rise*. HarperCollins.

Keppley, W. (2017). A lesson in kindness. In A. Newmark & A. Kajitani (Eds.), *Inspiration for Teachers* (pp. 192–194). Chicken Soup for the Soul.

Kim, B. S. K. (2010). Client motivation and multicultural counseling. *The Counseling Psychologist*, 39(2), 267–275.

Klein, H. J., Lount, R. B., Jr., Park, H. M., & Linford, B. J. (2020). When goals are known: The effects of audience relative status on goal commitment and performance. *Journal of Applied Psychology*, 105(4), 372–389.

Knoll, L. J., Leung, J. T., Foulkes, L., & Blakemore, S. J. (2017). Age-related differences in social influence on risk perception depend on the direction of influence. *Journal of Adolescence*, 60, 53–63.

Knowles, T. (2021). First Person: Juggling through a teacher education program. *Phi Delta Kappan*, 103(2), 58–59.

Kohn, A. (1992). *No Contest: The Case against Competition*. Houghton Mifflin Harcourt.

Kreausukon, P., Gellert, P., Lippke, S., & Schwarzer, R. (2012). Planning and self-efficacy can increase fruit and vegetable consumption: A randomized controlled trial. *Journal of Behavioral Medicine*, 35(4), 443–451.

Kristof, N. D. (2012, January 22). How Mrs. Grady transformed Olly Neal. *New York Times*.

Kuzma, C. (2019, December 11). 8 unusual things Diljeet Taylor does that make her a top NCAA coach. *Runner's World*. Retrieved from www.runnersworld.com/health-injuries/a30191488/why-diljeet-taylor-is-a-top-ncaa-coach/

Ladson-Billings, G. (1995). Toward a theory of culturally relevant pedagogy. *American Educational Research Journal*, 32(3), 465–491.

Lam, C. B., McHale, S. M., & Crouter, A. C. (2014). Time with peers from middle childhood to late adolescence: Developmental course and adjustment correlates. *Child Development*, 85(4), 1677–1693.

Lampert, M., Rittenhouse, P., & Crumbaugh, C. (1996). Agreeing to disagree: Developing sociable mathematical discourse. In D. R. Olson & N. Torrance (Eds.), *The Handbook of Education and Human Development* (pp. 731–764). Blackwell.

Lareau, A. (1989). *Home Advantage: Social Class and Parental Intervention in Elementary Education*. Falmer Press.

Lareau, A. (2003). *Unequal Childhoods: Class, Race, and Family Life*. University of California Press.

Lareau, A., & Calarco, J. (2012). Class, cultural capital, and institutions: The case of families and schools. In H. Markus & S. T. Fiske (Eds.), *Facing Social Class* (pp. 61–86). Russell Sage Foundation.

Laurin, K. (2016). Interpersonal influences on goals: Current and future directions for goal contagion research. *Social and Personality Psychology Compass*, 10(11), 668–678.

Lee, C. D. (1993). *Signifying as a Scaffold for Literary Interpretation: The Pedagogical Implications of an African American Discourse Genre*. National Council of Teachers of English.

Lee, C. D. (1995). A culturally based cognitive apprenticeship: Teaching African American high school students skills in literary interpretation. *Reading Research Quarterly*, 30(4), 608–630.

Lee, H. S., & Anderson, J. R. (2013). Student learning: What has instruction got to do with it? *Annual Review of Psychology*, 64(1), 445–469.

Leonard, B. J., Skay, C. L., & Rheinberger, M. M. (1998). Self-management development in children and adolescents with diabetes: The role of maternal self-efficacy and conflict. *Journal of Pediatric Nursing*, 13(4), 224–233.

Leslie, S.-J., Cimpian, A., Meyer, M., & Freeland, E. (2015). Expectations of brilliance underlie gender distributions across academic disciplines. *Science*, 347(6219), 262.

Lewin, T. (2012, March 6). Black students face more discipline data suggests. *The New York Times*, Section A, Page 11. Retrieved from www.nytimes.com/2012/03/06/education/black-students-face-more-harsh-discipline-data-shows.html

Lewis, J., Ream, R., Bocian, K., Cardullo, R., Hammond, K., & Fast, L. (2012). Con cariño: Teacher caring, math self-efficacy, and math achievement among Hispanic English learners. *Teachers College Record*, 114(7), 1–42.

Lewis, M. (2004). Coach Fitz's management theory. *The New York Times Magazine*. Retrieved from www.nytimes.com/2004/03/28/magazine/coach-fitz-s-management-theory.html

Lewis, N. (2017). What if I'd dropped that class. In A. Newmark & A. Kajitani (Eds.), *Inspiration for Teachers* (pp. 185–188). Chicken Soup for the Soul.

Lin-Siegler, X., Ahn, J. N., Chen, J., Fang, F.-F. A., & Luna-Lucero, M. (2016). Even Einstein struggled: Effects of learning about great scientists' struggles on high school students' motivation to learn science. *Journal of Educational Psychology*, 108(3), 314–328.

Linnenbrink-Garcia, L., Pugh, K. J., Koskey, K. L. K., & Stewart, V. C. (2012). Developing conceptual understanding of natural selection: The role of interest, efficacy, and basic prior knowledge. *The Journal of Experimental Education*, 80(1), 45–68.

Locke, E. A., & Latham, G. P. (1990). *A Theory of Goal Setting and Task Performance*. Prentice-Hall.

Locke, E. A., & Latham, G. P. (2002). Building a practically useful theory of goal setting and task motivation: A 35-year odyssey. *American Psychologist*, 57(9), 705–717.

Locke, E. A., & Latham, G. P. (2006). New directions in goal-setting theory. *Current Direction in Psychological Science*, 15, 265–268.

Locke, E. A., & Latham, G. P. (2013). *New Developments In Goal Setting and Task Performance*. Routledge.

Locke, E. A., Latham, G. P., & Erez, M. (1988). The determinants of goal commitment. *The Academy of Management Review*, 13(1), 23–39.

Loeb, E. L., Kansky, J., Tan, J. S., Costello, M. A., & Allen, J. P. (2021). Perceived psychological control in early adolescence predicts lower levels of adaptation into mid-adulthood. *Child Development*, 92(2), e158–e172.

Lopez, N. (2016). *The Bridge to Brilliance*. Viking.

Luszczynska, A., Tryburc, M., & Schwarzer, R. (2007). Improving fruit and vegetable consumption: A self-efficacy intervention compared with a combined self-efficacy and planning intervention. *Health Education Research*, 22(5), 630–638.

MacGillivray, L., & Curwen, M. S. (2007). Tagging as a social literacy practice. *Journal of Adolescent & Adult Literacy*, 50(5), 354–369.

Mali, T. (2012). *What Teachers Make: In Praise of the Greatest Job in the World*. G. P. Putnam's Sons.

Maloney, E. A., Ramirez, G., Gunderson, E. A., Levine, S. C., & Beilock, S. L. (2015). Intergenerational effects of parents' math anxiety on children's math achievement and anxiety. *Psychological Science*, 26(9), 1480–1488.

Mar, R. A., & Oatley, K. (2008). The function of fiction is the abstraction and simulation of social experience. *Perspectives on Psychological Science*, 3(3), 173–192.

Marks, R., & Allegrante, J. P. (2005). A review and synthesis of research evidence for self-efficacy-enhancing interventions for reducing chronic disability: Implications for health education practice (Part II). *Health Promotion Practice*, 6(2), 148–156.

Markus, P. (2017). *Inside my Pencil: Teaching Poetry in the Detroit Public Schools.* Dzanc Books.

Martin, A. J., & Elliot, A. J. (2016). The role of personal best (PB) goal setting in students' academic achievement gains. *Learning and Individual Differences*, 45, 222–227.

Martin, M. J., McCarthy, B., Conger, R. D., Gibbons, F. X., Simons, R. L., Cutrona, C. E., & Brody, G. H. (2011). The enduring significance of racism: Discrimination and delinquency among Black American youth. *Journal of Research on Adolescence*, 21(3), 662–676.

McCourt, F. (2005). *Teacher Man.* Scribner.

McGinley, W., & Kamberelis, G. (1996). Maniac Magee and Ragtime Tumpie: Children negotiating self and world through reading and writing. *Research in the Teaching of English*, 30(1), 75–113.

McGrew, K. (2011). A review of class-based theories of student resistance in education: Mapping the origins and influence of learning to labor by Paul Willis. *Review of Educational Research*, 81(2), 234–266.

McKinney, C. (2017). The weight of labels. In A. Newmark & A. Kajitani (Eds.), *Inspiration for Teachers* (pp. 256–258). Chicken Soup for the Soul.

Mirón, L. F., & Lauria, M. (1998). Student voice as agency: Resistance and accommodation in inner-city schools. *Anthropology & Education Quarterly*, 29(2), 189–213.

Mistry, J., & Kiyama, F. (2021). Navigating marginalization and invisibility as Asian Americans in the US. *American Psychologist*, 76(4), 582–595.

Moje, E. B. (2000). "To be part of the story": The literacy practices of gangsta adolescents. *Teachers College Record*, 102(3), 651–690.

Monzó, L. D., & Rueda, R. (2009). Passing for English fluent: Latino immigrant children masking language proficiency. *Anthropology & Education Quarterly*, 40(1), 20–40.

Morisano, D. (2013). Goal setting in the academic arena. In E. A. Locke & G. P. Latham (Eds.), *New Developments in Goal Setting and Task Performance* (pp. 495–506). Routledge.

Morisano, D., Hirsh, J. B., Peterson, J. B., Pihl, R. O., & Shore, B. M. (2010). Setting, elaborating, and reflecting on personal goals improves academic performance. *Journal of Applied Psychology*, 95(2), 255–264.

Moulard, J. G., Kroff, M., Pounders, K., & Ditt, C. (2019). The role of suspense in gaming: Inducing consumers' game enjoyment. *Journal of Interactive Advertising*, 19(3), 219–235.

Muñoz, J. P. (2007). Culturally responsive caring in occupational therapy. *Occupational Therapy International*, 14(4), 256–280.

Murayama, K., & Elliot, A. J. (2012). The competition–performance relation: A meta-analytic review and test of the opposing processes model of competition and performance. *Psychological Bulletin*, 138(6), 1035–1070.

Murphy, P. K., & Alexander, P. A. (2002). What counts? The predictive powers of subject-matter knowledge, strategic processing, and interest in domain-specific performance. *Journal of Experimental Education*, 70(3), 197.

Nadal, K. L. (2011). The Racial and Ethnic Microaggressions Scale (REMS): Construction, reliability, and validity. *Journal of Counseling Psychology*, 58(4), 470–480.

National Assessment of Educational Progress (2019). *NAEP Report Card: Mathematics*. Retrieved from www.nationsreportcard.gov

Neu, T. W., Baum, S. M., & Cooper, C. R. (2004). Talent development in science: A unique tale of one student's journey. *The Journal of Secondary Gifted Education*, 16(1), 30–36.

Niederle, M., & Vesterlund, L. (2011). Gender and competition. *Annual Review of Economics*, 3(1), 601–630.

O'Neil, H. F., Abedi, J., Miyoshi, J., & Mastergeorge, A. (2005). Monetary incentives for low-stakes tests. *Educational Assessment*, 10(3), 185–208.

O'Neil, H. F., Sugrue, B., & Baker, E. L. (1995/1996). Effects of motivational interventions on the National Assessment of Educational Progress mathematics performance. *Educational Assessment*, 3(2), 135–157.

O'Reilly, T., Wang, Z., & Sabatini, J. (2019). How much knowledge is too little? When a lack of knowledge becomes a barrier to comprehension. *Psychological Science*, 30(9), 1344–1351.

Okoroafor, C. (2016). All the African influences in Beyoncés visual album, Lemonade, explained. Retrieved from https://venturesafrica.com/features/the-african-influences-in-beyonces-lemonade-album-explained/

Olson, S. (2004). *Count Down: Six Kids Vie for Glory at the World's Toughest Math Competition*. Houghton Mifflin.

Owens, J. (2013). *Confessions of a Bad Teacher*. Sourcebooks.

Pappas, A. (2019). Hearing the "Bo Diddley Beat" in everything. Retrieved from https://flypaper.soundfly.com/discover/hearing-the-bo-diddley-beat-in-everything/

Parkhouse, H., Lu, C. Y., & Massaro, V. R. (2019). Multicultural education professional development: A review of the literature. *Review of Educational Research*, 89(3), 416–458.

Patall, E. A., Cooper, H., & Robinson, J. C. (2008). The effects of choice on intrinsic motivation and related outcomes: A meta-analysis of research findings. *Psychological Bulletin*, 134(2), 270–300.

Paunesku, D., Walton, G. M., Romero, C., Smith, E. N., Yeager, D. S., & Dweck, C. S. (2015). Mind-set interventions are a scalable treatment for academic underachievement. *Psychological Science*, 26(6), 784–793.

Pearson, J. (2006). Personal control, self-efficacy in sexual negotiation, and contraceptive risk among adolescents: The role of gender. *Sex Roles*, 54(9), 615–625.

Pennebaker, J., & Chung, C. (2012). Expressive writing: Connections for physical and mental health. In H. Friedman (Ed.), *Oxford Handbook of Health Psychology*. Oxford.

Perry, S. (2011). *Push Has Come to Shove*. Crown.

Plaut, V. C., Thomas, K. M., & Goren, M. J. (2009). Is multiculturalism or color blindness better for minorities? *Psychological Science*, 20(4), 444–446.

Plaut, V. C., Thomas, K. M., Hurd, K., & Romano, C. A. (2018). Do color blindness and multiculturalism remedy or foster discrimination and racism? *Current Directions in Psychological Science*, 27(3), 200–206.

Powell, C. (1995). *My American Journey*. Random House.

Programme for International Student Assessment (2020). *Do students learn in cooperative or competitive environments?* Retrieved from www.oecd-ilibrary.org

Pugh, K. J. (2020). *Transformative Science Education*. Teachers College Press.

Pugh, K. J., & Bergin, D. A. (2005). The effect of schooling on students' out-of-school experience. *Educational Researcher*, 34(9), 15–23.

Pugh, K. J., Bergstrom, C. M., & Spencer, B. (2017). Profiles of transformative engagement: Identification, description, and relation to learning and instruction. *Science Education*, 101(3), 369–398.

Pugh, K. J., Bergstrom, C. M., Heddy, B. C., & Krob, K. E. (2017). Supporting deep engagement: The teaching for transformative experiences in science (TTES) model. *Journal of Experimental Education*, 85(4), 629–657.

Pugh, K. J., Linnenbrink-Garcia, L., Koskey, K. L. K., Stewart, V. C., & Manzey, C. (2010). Teaching for transformative experiences and conceptual change: A case study and evaluation of a high school biology teacher's experience. *Cognition and Instruction*, 28(3), 273–316.

Purcell-Gates, V. (1995). *Other People's Words*. Harvard.

Raicu, L. (2017). Doing something right. In A. Newmark & A. Kajitani (Eds.), *Inspiration for Teachers* (pp. 13–15). Chicken Soup for the Soul.

Ramirez, G., & Beilock, S. L. (2011). Writing about testing worries boosts exam performance in the classroom. *Science*, 331(6014), 211.

Reeve, J. (2009). Why teachers adopt a controlling motivating style toward students and how they can become more autonomy supportive. *Educational Psychologist*, 44(3), 159–175.

Reeve, J., & Cheon, S. H. (2021). Autonomy-supportive teaching: Its malleability, benefits, and potential to improve educational practice. *Educational Psychologist*, 56(1), 54–77.

Reeve, J., & Deci, E. L. (1996). Elements of the competitive situation that affect intrinsic motivation. *Personality and Social Psychology Bulletin*, 22(1), 24–33.

Rege, M., Hanselman, P., Solli, I. F., Dweck, C. S., Ludvigsen, S., Bettinger, E., Crosnoe, R., Muller, C., Walton, G., Duckworth, A., & Yeager, D. S. (2021). How can we inspire nations of learners? An investigation of growth mindset and challenge-seeking in two countries. *American Psychologist*, 76(5), 755–767.

Renkl, A., Mandl, H., & Gruber, H. (1996). Inert knowledge: Analyses and remedies. *Educational Psychologist*, 31(2), 115–121.

Renninger, K. A., & Hidi, S. (2011). Revisiting the conceptualization, measurement, and generation of interest. *Educational Psychologist*, 46(3), 168–184.

Reusser, K. (1988). Problem solving beyond the logic of things: Contextual effects on understanding and solving word problems. *Instructional Science*, 17(4), 309–338.

Rios-Aguilar, C., Kiyama, J. M., Gravitt, M., & Moll, L. C. (2011). Funds of knowledge for the poor and forms of capital for the rich? A capital approach to examining funds of knowledge. *Theory and Research in Education*, 9(2), 163–184.

Ripley, A. (2013). *The Smartest Kids in the World*. Simon & Schuster.

Rivas-Drake, D., Seator, E. K., Markstrom, C., Quintana, S., Syed, M., Lee, R. M., Schwartz, S. J., Umaña-Taylor, A. J., French, S., Yip, T., & Ethnic and Racial Identity in the 21st Century Study Group. (2014). Ethnic and racial identity in adolescence: Implications for psychosocial, academic and health outcomes. *Child Development*, 85(1), 40–57.

Robinson, C. D., Scott, W., & Gottfried, M. A. (2019). Taking it to the next level: A field experiment to improve instructor-student relationships in college. *AERA Open*, 5(1).

Rohde, A., Townley-O'Neill, K., Trendall, K., Worrall, L., & Cornwell, P. (2012). A comparison of client and therapist goals for people with aphasia: A qualitative exploratory study. *Aphasiology*, 26(10), 1298–1315.

Roorda, D. L., & Koomen, H. M. Y. (2021). Student–teacher relationships and students' externalizing and internalizing behaviors: A cross-lagged study in secondary education. *Child Development*, 92(1), 174–188.

Roorda, D. L., Koomen, H. M. Y., Spilt, J. L., & Oort, F. J. (2011). The influence of affective teacher–student relationships on students' school engagement and achievement. *Review of Educational Research*, 81(4), 493–529.

Rosenbloom, S. R., & Way, N. (2004). Experiences of discrimination among African American, Asian American, and Latino adolescents in an urban high school. *Youth & Society*, 35(4), 420–451.

Rosenfield, S. (2018). *Mastering Stand-up*. Chicago Review Press.

Ryan, R. M. (2015). Foreword. In A. Poulsen, J. Ziviani, & M. Cuskelly (Eds.), *Goal Setting and Motivation in Therapy: Engaging Children and Parents* (pp. 17–20). Jessica Kingsley.

Ryan, R. M., & Deci, E. L. (2000). Self-determination theory and the facilitation of intrinsic motivation, social development, and well-being. *American Psychologist*, 55(1), 68–78.

Ryan, R. M., & Deci, E. L. (2020). Intrinsic and extrinsic motivation from a self-determination theory perspective: Definitions, theory, practices, and future directions. *Contemporary Educational Psychology*, 61.

Ryan, R. M., Lynch, M. F., Vansteenkiste, M., & Deci, E. L. (2011). Motivation and autonomy in counseling, psychotherapy, and behavior change: A look at theory and practice. *The Counseling Psychologist*, 39(2), 193–260.

Sakiz, G., Pape, S. J., & Hoy, A. W. (2012). Does perceived teacher affective support matter for middle school students in mathematics classrooms? *Journal of School Psychology*, 50(2), 235–255.

Schaeffer, M. W., Rozek, C. S., Berkowitz, T., Levine, S. C., & Beilock, S. L. (2018). Disassociating the relation between parents' math anxiety and children's math achievement: Long-term effects of a math app intervention. *Journal of Experimental Psychology: General*, 147(12), 1782–1790.

Schank, R. C. (1979). Interestingness: Controlling inferences. *Artificial Intelligence*, 12(3), 273–297.

Scharf, M., & Goldner, L. (2018) "If you really love me, you will do/be …": Parental psychological control and its implications for children's adjustment. *Developmental Review*, 49, 16–30.

Schellong, M. (2021, November 24). Confederation of Michigan Tribal Education Departments introduces first-ever Indigenous resource guide for state's K-12 schools. WKAR Public Media. Retrieved from www.wkar.org/wkar-news/2021-11-24/confederation-of-michigan-tribal-education-departments-introduces-first-ever-indigenous-resource-guide-for-states-k-12-schools?fbclid=IwAR0MdOOdnAYGrz5K9z3YJhVCgSPesnUJvnZBlMpL1WjjWBvMtmGrN1tKB6w

Schleef, D. (2000). "That's a good question!" Exploring motivations for law and business school choice. *Sociology of Education*, 73(3), 155–174.

Schmitt, M. T., Branscombe, N. R., Postmes, T., & Garcia, A. (2014). The consequences of perceived discrimination for psychological well-being: A meta-analytic review. *Psychological Bulletin*, 140(4), 921–948.

Schoenfeld, A. (1989). Teaching mathematical thinking and problem solving. In L. Resnick & L. Klopfer (Eds.), *Toward the Thinking Curriculum* (pp. 83–103). Association for Supervision and Curriculum Development.

Schutz, P. A., Crowder, K. C., & White, V. E. (2001). The development of a goal to become a teacher. *Journal of Educational Psychology*, 93(2), 299–308.

Schwinger, M., Wirthwein, L., Lemmer, G., & Steinmayr, R. (2014). Academic self-handicapping and achievement: A meta-analysis. *Journal of Educational Psychology*, 106(3), 744–761.

Sheeran, P., Maki, A., Montanaro, E., Avishai-Yitshak, A., Bryan, A., Klein, W. M. P., Miles, E., & Rothman, A. J. (2016). The impact of changing attitudes, norms, and self-efficacy on health-related intentions and behavior: A meta-analysis. *Health Psychology*, 35(11), 1178–1188.

Shirk, S. R., Karver, M. S., & Brown, R. (2011). The alliance in child and adolescent psychotherapy. *Psychotherapy*, 48(1), 17–24.

Sirin, S. R., Rogers-Sirin, L., Cressen, J., Gupta, T., Ahmed, S. F., & Novoa, A. D. (2015). Discrimination-related stress effects on the development of internalizing symptoms among Latino adolescents. *Child Development*, 86(3), 709–725.

Sjödin, S. (2015). Negotiating learner autonomy: A case study on the autonomy of a learner with high-functioning autism. *Nordic Journal of Studies in Educational Policy*, 2015(2), 86–94.

Slavin, R. E. (2010). Can financial incentives enhance educational outcomes? Evidence from international experiments. *Educational Research Review*, 5, 68–80.

Smith, E. B. (1995). Anchored in our literature: Students responding to African American literature. *Language Arts*, 72, 571–574.

Smitherman, G. (2000). *Black Talk: Words and Phrases from the Hood to the Amen Corner* (revised ed.). Houghton Mifflin.

Song, H., Kim, J., Tenzek, K. E., & Lee, K. M. (2013). The effects of competition and competitiveness upon intrinsic motivation in exergames. *Computers in Human Behavior*, 29(4), 1702–1708.

Soto, A., Smith, T. B., Griner, D., Domenech Rodríguez, M., & Bernal, G. (2018). Cultural adaptations and therapist multicultural competence: Two meta-analytic reviews. *Journal of Clinical Psychology*, 74(11), 1907–1923.

Spears-Bunton, L. A. (1990). Welcome to my house: African American and European American students' responses to Virginia Hamilton's House of Dies Drear. *The Journal of Negro Education*, 59(4), 566–576.

Spencer, M. B., Noll, E., & Cassidy, E. (2005). Monetary incentives in support of academic achievement. *Evaluation Review*, 29(3), 199–222.

Stefanou, C. R., Perencevich, K. C., DiCintio, M., & Turner, J. C. (2004). Supporting autonomy in the classroom: Ways teachers encourage student decision making and ownership. *Educational Psychologist*, 39(2), 97–110.

Stein, G. L., Supple, A. J., Huq, N., Dunbar, A. S., & Prinstein, M. J. (2016). A longitudinal examination of perceived discrimination and depressive symptoms in ethnic minority youth: The roles of attributional style, positive ethnic/racial affect, and emotional reactivity. *Developmental Psychology*, 52(2), 259–271.

Steketee, A., Williams, M. T., Valencia, B. T., Printz, D., & Hooper, L. M. (2021). Racial and language microaggressions in the school ecology. *Perspectives on Psychological Science*, 16(5), 1075–1098.

Stevens, W. E. (2021). Blackfishing on Instagram: Influencing and the commodification of Black urban aesthetics. *Social Media + Society*, 7(3).

Storage, D., Charlesworth, T. E. S., Banaji, M. R., & Cimpian, A. (2020). Adults and children implicitly associate brilliance with men more than women. *Journal of Experimental Social Psychology*, 90, 104020.

Sue, D. W., Capodilupo, C. M., Torino, G. C., Bucceri, J. M., Holder, A. M. B., Nadal, K. L., & Esquilin, M. (2007). Racial microaggressions in everyday life: Implications for clinical practice. *American Psychologist*, 62(4), 271–286.

Sue, S., Zane, N., Nagayama Hall, G. C., & Berger, L. K. (2008). The case for cultural competency in psychotherapeutic interventions. *Annual Review of Psychology*, 60(1), 525–548.

Sullo, B. (2009). *The Motivated Student*. ASCD.

Sundararajan, N., & Adesope, O. (2020). Keep it coherent: A meta-analysis of the seductive details effect. *Educational Psychology Review*, 32(3), 707–734.

Taing, V. (2009). Boy lifts book: librarian changes boy's life [NPR Morning Edition, interview from StoryCorps]. Retrieved from www.npr.org/templates/story/story.php?storyId=113357239

Tauer, J. M., & Harackiewicz, J. M. (1999). Winning isn't everything: Competition, achievement orientation, and intrinsic motivation. *Journal of Experimental Social Psychology*, 35(3), 209–238.

This American Life (2013). Harper High School - Part one. WBEZ Chicago. Retrieved from www.thisamericanlife.org/487/harper-high-school-part-one

Thompson, J. (2020). *I Came as a Shadow*. Henry Holt.

Tobias, S. (1994). Interest, prior knowledge, and learning. *Review of Educational Research*, 64(1), 37–54.

Todd, A. S., Street, S. J., Zivian, J., Byrne, N. M., & Hills, A. P. (2015). Overweight and obese adolescent girls: The importance of promoting sensible eating and activity behaviors from the start of the adolescent period. *International Journal of Environmental Research and Public Health*, 12(2), 2306–2329.

Tomova, L., Andrews, J. L., & Blakemore, S.-J. (2021). The importance of belonging and the avoidance of social risk taking in adolescence. *Developmental Review*, 61, 100981.

Tosto, M. G., Asbury, K., Mazzocco, M. M. M., Petrill, S. A., & Kovas, Y. (2016). From classroom environment to mathematics achievement: The mediating role of self-perceived ability and subject interest. *Learning and Individual Differences*, 50, 260–269.

Trayes, J., Harré, N., & Overall, N. C. (2012). A youth performing arts experience: Psychological experiences, recollections, and the desire to do it again. *Journal of Adolescent Research*, 27(2), 155–182.

Tryon, G. S. (2018). Goals and psychotherapy research. In D. Law & M. Cooper (Eds.), *Working with Goals in Psychotherapy and Counselling* (pp. 87–109). Oxford.

Tryon, G. S., Birch, S. E., & Verkuilen, J. (2018). Meta-analyses of the relation of goal consensus and collaboration to psychotherapy outcome. *Psychotherapy*, 55(4), 372–383.

Turner, E., & Strawhun, B. (2004/2005). With math, it's like you have more defence. *Rethinking Schools*, 19(1).

Turner, J. C., Warzon, K. B., & Christensen, A. (2011). Motivating mathematics learning. *American Educational Research Journal*, 48(3), 718–762.

Ukpokodu, O. (2011). How do I teach mathematics in a culturally responsive way? *Multicultural Education*, 18(3), 47–56.

Ulichny, P. (1996). Cultures in conflict. *Anthropology & Education Quarterly*, 27(3), 331–364.

Umaña-Taylor, A. J., Quintana, S. M., Lee, R. M., Cross Jr, W. E., Rivas-Drake, D., Schwartz, S. J., Syed, M., Yip, T., Seaton, E., & Ethnic and Racial Identity in the 21st Century Study Group (2014). Ethnic and racial identity during adolescence and into young adulthood: An integrated conceptualization. *Child Development*, 85(1), 21–39.

US Surgeon General (2021). *Protecting Youth Mental Health*. Department of Health and Human Services.

Usher, E. L. (2009). Sources of middle school students' self-efficacy in mathematics: A qualitative investigation. *American Educational Research Journal*, 46(1), 275–314.

Usher, E. L., & Pajares, F. (2008). Sources of self-efficacy in school: Critical review of the literature and future directions. *Review of Educational Research*, 78(4), 751–796.

Vandereycken, W., & Vansteenkiste, M. (2009). Let eating disorder patients decide: Providing choice may reduce early drop-out from inpatient treatment. *European Eating Disorders Review*, 17(3), 177–183.

VanEtten, L., Briggs, M., DeWitt, J., Mansfield, C., & Kaeding, C. (2021). The implementation of therapeutic alliance in the rehabilitation of an elite pediatric athlete with Salter-Harris fracture. *International Journal of Sports Physical Therapy*, 16(2), 539–551.

Vansteenkiste, M., & Deci, E. L. (2003). Competitively contingent rewards and intrinsic motivation: Can losers remain motivated? *Motivation and Emotion*, 27(4), 273–299.

Venturo-Conerly, K. E., Fitzpatrick, O. M., Horn, R. L., Ugueto, A. M., & Weisz, J. R. (2022). Effectiveness of youth psychotherapy delivered remotely: A meta-analysis. *American Psychologist*, 77(1), 71–84.

Vigneron, P. (2013, Feb). Dominatrix. *Outside Magazine*, 42–48. Retrieved from www.outsideonline.com/1870301/fastest-woman-planet

Wade, S. E., Schraw, G., Buxton, W. M., & Hayes, M. T. (1993). Seduction of the strategic reader: Effects of interest on strategies and recall. *Reading Research Quarterly*, 28(2), 93–114.

Wang, M.-T., & Eccles, J. S. (2013). School context, achievement motivation, and academic engagement: A longitudinal study of school engagement using a multidimensional perspective. *Learning and Instruction*, 28, 12–23.

Wankat, P. C. (2005). Undergraduate student competitions. *Journal of Engineering Education*, 94(3), 343–347.

Wankat, P. C. (2007). Survey of K-12 engineering-oriented student competitions. *International Journal of Engineering Education*, 23(1), 78–83.

Weinberg, R. (2010). Making goals effective: A primer for coaches. *Journal of Sport Psychology in Action*, 1(2), 57–65.

Wentzel, K. R. (1997). Student motivation in middle school: The role of perceived pedagogical caring. *Journal of Educational Psychology*, 89(3), 411–419.

Wentzel, K. R., Battle, A., Russell, S. L., & Looney, L. B. (2010). Social supports from teachers and peers as predictors of academic and social motivation. *Contemporary Educational Psychology*, 35(3), 193–202.

Wentzel, K. R., Tomback, R., Williams, A., & McNeish, D. (2019). Perceptions of competence, control, and belongingness over the transition to high school: A mixed-method study. *Contemporary Educational Psychology*, 56, 55–66.

Wesselmann, E. D., Cardoso, F. D., Slater, S., & Williams, K. D. (2012). To be looked at as though air: Civil attention matters. *Psychological Science*, 23(2), 166–168.

Wheeler, S. (2011). The significance of family culture for sports participation. *International Review for the Sociology of Sport*, 47(2), 235–252.

Whitehead, A. N. (1959, reprinted from 1929). The aims of education. *Daedalus*, 88(1), 192–205.

Winner, E. (1996). The rage to master: The decisive role of talent in the visual arts. In K. A. Ericsson (Ed.), *The Road to Excellence: The Acquisition of Expert Performance in the Arts and Sciences, Sports, and Games* (pp. 271–301). Erlbaum.

Woolley, M. E., Rose, R. A., Orthner, D. K., Akos, P. T., & Jones-Sanpei, H. (2013). Advancing academic achievement through career relevance in the middle grades: A longitudinal evaluation of CareerStart. *American Educational Research Journal*, 50(6), 1309–1335.

Yamawaki, N. (2021, Fall). Loving like Christ: An immigrant shares her journey to America and toward God. *Y Magazine*.

Yip, T., Cheah, C. S. L., Kiang, L., & Hall, G. C. N. (2021). Rendered invisible: Are Asian Americans a model or a marginalized minority? *American Psychologist*, 76(4), 575–581.

Zahorik, J. A. (1996). Elementary and secondary teachers' reports of how they make learning interesting. *Elementary School Journal*, 96(5), 551–564.

Zakrajsek, R. A., Fisher, L. A., & Martin, S. B. (2017). Certified athletic trainers' understanding and use of sport psychology in their practice. *Journal of Applied Sport Psychology*, 29(2), 215–233.

Zee, M., & Koomen, H. M. Y. (2016). Teacher self-efficacy and its effects on classroom processes, student academic adjustment, and teacher well-being: A synthesis of 40 years of research. *Review of Educational Research*, 86(4), 981–1015.

Zee, M., Rudasill, K. M., & Bosman, R. J. (2021). A cross-lagged study of students' motivation, academic achievement, and relationships with teachers from kindergarten to 6th grade. *Journal of Educational Psychology*, 113(6), 1208–1226.

Zhang, L. (2016). Is inquiry-based science teaching worth the effort? *Science & Education*, 25(7), 897–915.

Zhang, T., Chen, A., Yli-Piipari, S., Loflin, J., Wells, S., Schweighardt, R., Moennich, K., Hong, D., & Ennis, C. D. (2016). Prior knowledge determines interest in learning in physical education: A structural growth model perspective. *Learning and Individual Differences*, 51, 132–140.

Zuroff, D. C., Koestner, R., Moskowitz, D. S., McBride, C., & Bagby, R. M. (2012). Therapist's autonomy support and patient's self-criticism predict motivation during brief treatments for depression. *Journal of Social and Clinical Psychology*, 31(9), 903–932.

Index

For Product Safety Concerns and Information please contact our EU
representative GPSR@taylorandfrancis.com
Taylor & Francis Verlag GmbH, Kaufingerstraße 24, 80331 München, Germany